Hormones: A Woman's Self Help Guide to Natural Balance

ABIOLA O. OLADOKE, Ph.D.

To all Women, past, present and future.

This book is not intended to provide traditional allopathic medical advice. Readers are encouraged to seek medical advice from their health care practitioners regarding matters of health and wellness. This publication provides natural wellness tips and information beneficial to the general populace. It is not designed for individualized treatment protocols; for that, please visit with your health care provider. The author and publisher specifically disclaim any liability or risk which is incurred as a consequence, directly or indirectly, of the use and application of any of the contents of this work.

FIRST EDITION

ISBN: 978-0982003114

hp Health-centric Publications

Hormones: A Woman's Self-Help Guide to Natural Balance

CONTENTS

ACKNOWLEDGMENTS

There are many people who have made it possible for this book to happen. First I want to thank the DIVINE for grace, mercy, wisdom and application of knowledge. I want to thank the wonderful women who trust me with their natural health and listened to my coaching. The protocols in this book would only be theories if not for you all. Thank you. My gratitude to my parents, who have been my supporters even when they had no idea what I was doing. My gratitude to my friends who combed the book for fat finger errors and offered support on many levels than I can list. Deep appreciation to my lovely model, Christina Blanco and her mother, Ophelia Blanco who opened her home to me for the photos and many more things that I will forever be grateful for. A big "thank you" to Paula Martinez who attended one of my information seminars at the behest of "Aunt Jerry" and has been spreading the word. Lastly, to all the believers who know that Nature offers answers, even those we don't quite like but are open to receiving, thank you for supporting the cause for natural health care and prevention.

Many blessings.

Introduction

Let me begin by saying thank you for purchasing my work. I am very grateful.

I began my journey to endocrinally balanced diet in 2005. At the time, I was sick with many health problems and at a loss about what to do. Modern medicine did not have any favorable answers for me so I turned to Mother Earth. I figured, I am from Her, She should have the answers and She did.

After much research, studying, and experience with myself, I found the answers in Nature. I didn't stop with personal experiments, I returned to school to study various alternative approaches to wellness and my ill-health created the zeal to recover as well as a new career path. I went from helping my own body recover and stay well to assisting other men and women achieve and maintain the same. In this book, my focus is solely on women for two reasons: first, the full story needs to be told from a woman's perspective and second, I gotta take care of my ladies because we take care of everybody else and forget about ourselves.

What we eat and do determine how well we feel and look. From the emotional standpoint, humans have many combinations and permutations of hormones coursing through our veins daily. These hormones determine how well or how awful we feel and they are highly influenced by what we put in our mouths, our work, outlook on life and much more.

In the following pages, I have provided some information about the endocrine system and how what we eat influences this system. After the scientific information about hormones and emotions, I dive right into the fun part of herbs, food and awesome recipes you can start to enjoy so you can balance your emotions and some aroma medicine recipes. I also added some scripts from my practice to help you subconsciously handle your emotions and release stress in the comfort of your home. I encourage you to record the scripts in your own voice and listen to them at will. Lastly, I included some meridian exercises to tone and improve the function of the endocrine organs.

You can start from the Food Facts section and the recipes if you like or you can read all the research information first. If you want to know why it is important to eat a plant based diet, start at the beginning. If you are already set to correct your emotional imbalance and know that food is a great way to get there, dive right in at the Food Facts and Recipes. But please return to the scientific stuff because it will help you appreciate your decision to take care of your hormonal health.

Understanding Hormones in Women

Okay, before we get to the recipes and natural methods that support hormonal and emotional balance, I want to take some time to share with you how our bodies make and use hormones and what this means for our health and wellness as women. This chapter shares basic information about the endocrine system, some information about hormone creation and regulation, causes of hormone imbalance, effects of hormone imbalance, and treating hormone imbalance naturally. This chapter is a little technical but you need to understand what is happening. Don't worry, after this chapter, we are on to the fun information: how to eat to balance hormones and our emotions. Yeah!

Now, we all know that organs, nerves, muscles, tendons, tissues, bones, veins, capillaries, arteries, cells, and chemicals to mention a few comprise the human body. The functions of the different parts of the human body have been classified into systems and they are: the nervous, endocrine, skeletal, respiratory, circulatory/cardiovascular, immune, digestive, urinary, reproductive, muscular, and lymphatic systems. The systems work together to ensure the human body can function at its optimal. It's like an orchestra that can't play good music if the cellist and the violinist are not working. The human brain plays an integral role in the functioning of all the systems; the circulatory/cardiovascular system is also importantly connected to the other systems and some of the systems are directly connected to the heart while others are not. From the many systems in the human body, the endocrine system secretes hormones that regulate reproductive functions in men and women; the secretion of hormones is one of the many responsibilities of the endocrine system, it plays a role in how the liver, kidneys, lungs and heart work, for example. The endocrine system comprise the hypothalamus, pituitary gland (anterior and posterior lobes), pineal gland, thyroid gland, parathyroid glands, thymus gland, adrenal glands, pancreatic islets, the ovaries, and the testes.

Current biological researches provide information about the roles and functions of the organs that comprise the endocrine system. The hypothalamus secretes several releasing and inhibiting hormones; mainly corticotrophin (ACTH), thyrotropin or thyroid stimulating hormone (TSH), follicle-stimulating hormone (FSH), luteinizing hormone (LH), prolactin (PRL), and somatotropin (STH). human chorionic gonadotropin (hCG), and (growth hormone) (GH). These hormones act on the different cells in the pituitary gland's anterior lobe and they also have roles in the production of antidiuretic hormone (ADH) and oxytocin (which has a role in childbirth and milk production). The functioning of the hypothalamus directly influences the actions of the pituitary's anterior and posterior lobes in their secretion, stimulation, and storage of hormones. The anterior lobe of the pituitary gland secretes and stores ACTH, TSH, FSH, LH, PRL, and STH, while the posterior lobe of the pituitary gland secretes and stores ADH and oxytocin. The pineal gland secretes melatonin, which affects the body's biological clock; it also influences the overall level of sexual activity and the reproductive cycles. The thyroid gland secretes thyroxine and triidothyronine, which have roles in the control of growth, development and metabolism. The parathyroid gland secretes parathyroid hormone that increases blood levels of calcium ions as needed.

The thymus gland secretes thymosin which influences immunity. The adrenal glands, further classified as the cortex and the medulla, have different roles. The adrenal cortex secrete cortisol, which affects the metabolism of glucose, and aldosterone, which conserves sodium; the adrenal medulla secrete epinephrine, norepinephrine. The adrenal medulla's secretions interact with the nervous system through the sympathetic nerves, to assist the body with adjustments of organ activities, especially when the body is experiencing stress or excitement.

The pancreatic islets secrete insulin, which lowers blood levels of glucose, glucagon, which raises blood level of glucose, and somatostatin, which influences the metabolism of carbohydrates. The ovaries secrete a group of hormones called estrogen and progesterone; these hormones maintain the sex organs and influence sexual activities. The testes secrete androgens, including testosterone, which serve the same roles as the hormones secreted by the ovaries, the ovaries are the female gonads and the testes are the male gonads.

In women, the reproductive system comprise the ovaries, oviducts, uterus, cervix, vagina and breasts. Hormones of the ovaries, oviducts and uterus are stimulated by the secretion of the follicle-stimulating hormone and luteinizing hormone in the pituitary gland; the pituitary gland is prompted by the signals from the hypothalamus. For proper reproductive hormone secretion and stimulation in women, the hypothalamus and pituitary gland need to secrete the follicle-stimulating and luteinizing hormones so that the follicles in the ovaries can be stimulated to create and release an egg in preparation for fertilization; the endometrial lining within the uterus is also stimulated to thicken in anticipation of egg cleavage, should fertilization occur. If there is no egg fertilization, the endometrial lining is shed in the form of a menstruation. The secretion, expectation of egg fertilization and shedding, if there is no fertilization, is termed the menstrual cycle.

The cycle begins with the stimulation of estrogen hormones that cause the uterine lining to thicken. At the time that the ovaries release an egg (ovulation), the follicle that released the egg begins to serve another purpose, it becomes corpus luteum and secretes progesterone. A disruption in the process of hormone secretion, which could be caused by a myriad of reasons, could prevent the ovaries from being stimulated to release an egg. When this happens, a woman is said to have an anovulatory cycle. Hormone disruption can also cause the ovaries to have incomplete egg releasing follicles thereby resulting in polycystic ovary syndrome. Research also show that the ovarian hormones have other functions besides ensuring proper reproductive system functioning; the ovarian hormones stimulate responses that ensure the rest of the body such as the lungs, heart, bone and blood vessels function normally. These hormones also greatly impact the normal functioning of the breasts, as can be noted when the pituitary gland secretes prolactin hormone in anticipation of childbirth.

So with all the basic information about hormones secretion, you can begin to gather that hormonal actions in the endocrine system require normal functioning of each part of the body to behave as it should. When hormonal processes are disrupted in one part of this system, the disruption delays responses and secretions in other parts and negatively impact a behavior or process that an individual may require. Warshowsky and Oumano explain that the hypothalamus needs to receive the signal from the limbic brain, telling it when to release hormones, in order for it to spur to action. Once the hypothalamus receives this signal, it sends gonadotropin-releasing hormone (GnRH) signal to the pituitary gland to secrete hormones and signal other parts in the endocrine system to secrete their hormones. The secretion of these hormones in the different parts of the endocrine system creates changes in their corresponding body parts. Since each part secretes different hormones and the receptor cells for each hormone differ, one hormone cannot occupy another hormone's target receptor.

Hormones have different functions in the body. The secretion of epinephrine and norepinephrine in the adrenal glands assist in the response to fear, stress, anxiety or excitement, while the secretion of estrogen influences the menstrual cycle. When the pituitary gland secretes follicle-stimulating hormone and luteinizing hormone, the ovarian hormones are created. The stimulation of the pituitary gland, the ovaries and the normal menstrual process regulates the cycle of hormones that impact the female reproductive system. The digestive system, mainly the liver, the kidneys, and the colon assist the reproductive system with regulating hormones by excreting the excess hormones from the body. Once ovarian hormones are created, any excess in the bloodstream is gathered by the liver and discarded via the bile duct into the colon where it is absorbed by soluble and insoluble fiber as waste and excreted with feces; excess hormones are also discarded through urination.

In the table on the next page, I provide a summary of endocrine functions. You will see that our glands work several miles a second to keep us upright; maybe you will then start to see why it is important to take excellent care of these glands. I believe in treating the body as the queen it truly is because I only have this one body and from past experience, it has whooped my butt severely when I failed to treat her as the queen she is.

Gland	Hormone Secreted	Functions
Pineal	Melatonin, Serotonin	Master gland responsible for maintaining our internal clock, regulates sleep and wake cycles (circadian rhythm); influences metabolism and sexual maturity; signals to pituitary when to secrete certain hormones; its complete function is still not known but I have found that working on it naturally helps all the other endocrine glands in their functionality.
Hypothalamus	Releases pre-factors for STH, TSH, LH, ACTH, MSH and PRL so the Pituitary can secrete them; this gland also secretes Oxytocin and Vasopressin to the pituitary	This gland tells the pituitary when to secrete and release the pituitary hormones; it also inhibits the secretion of these hormones.
Pituitary	Somatotropin (STH), Thyrotropin (TSH), Luteinizing Hormone (LH), Adrenocorticotropin (ACTH), Follicle-Stimulating Hormone (FSH), Vasopressin (ADH), Melanocyte Stimulating (MSH), Prolactin (PRL), Oxytocin	This gland releases all of the hormones mentioned in the left column and they work to regulate metabolism, protein synthesis, growth, thyroid gland, estrogen, progesterone, controls the ovaries and testes, adrenal function, blood pressure, function of the kidneys, and lactation.
Thyroid	Thyroxine, Calcitonin	Basal metabolism regulation, regulates growth and development
Parathyroid	Parathyroid hormone	Regulates the levels of phosporus and calcium in the blood
Thymus	Thymosin, Thymopoietin,	General immunity, cellular

Gland	Hormone Secreted	Functions
	Thymulin	immunity through the production of T-cells; influences the lymphatic glands; its other functions are still unknown. This gland atrophies as we get older and by puberty, the tissues becomes fat but it's still active.
Pancreas	Insulin, Glucagon	Helps to utilize glucose; regulates the blood sugar by secreting insulin and glucagon; insulin and glucagon have opposite actions
Adrenals	Glucocorticoids and mineralcorticoids (DHEA, cortisol, aldosterone, and others), estrogens, progesterone, androgens, epinephrine, norepinephrine	Control of blood sugar, increases the metabolism of protein and fat, influences carbohydrates, regulates potassium and sodium and water metabolism; supplements the actions of the ovaries, has anti-inflammatory and immunosupressive functions. Too much cortisol leads to Cushing's syndrome, too little cortisol leads to Addison's disease. Epinephrine is secreted to open airways to increase oxygen intake, increase heart rate and blood flow to the muscles in situations of stress, scare, anxiety or excitement (positive or negative); norepinephine helps to maintain normal activities, too much of it can cause high blood pressure
Ovaries	Estrogen, Progesterone, Relaxin	Work with hormones from the pituitary (luteinizing hormone and follicle-stimulating hormone) to control menstrual

Gland	Hormone Secreted	Functions
		cycle; produces inhibin, a protein that inhibits the release of follicle stimulating hormone, thus controlling egg development; regulates the development of female sexual organs, fertility and in maintaining pregnancy; relaxes the pelvic muscles and ligaments, regulates vaginal tissues, mood changes, bone density

Let's explore some causes of hormone imbalance in women. When hormones are created, they serve the purpose for which they were secreted and the same parts that secreted them work with the liver and the kidneys to regulate the hormones for proper excretion, to prevent excess secretion and stimulation. In instances where one part does not secrete the hormone it is supposed to or where one part continuously secrete and release one or more hormones, an imbalance of hormones in the bloodstream can occur; if the liver and kidneys are unable to successfully excrete the excess hormones because of problems that may be existent in the digestive or urinary system, the excess hormones are reabsorbed into the bloodstream and recirculated. This leads to hormone imbalance problems which could be over- or under-production of some hormones over others.

Several studies show there are many causes of hormone imbalance in women. These causes are continuous stress, emotional imbalance, poor nutrition, lack of exercise, iatrogenic substances, pesticides, plastics, herbicides, preservatives, and other chemicals that are used in food production. Studies also show that certain medications, such as birth control pills, cause or encourage hormone imbalance in women. The purpose of some birth control pills that contain one or more forms of estrogen is to prevent ovulation; anovulatory circle is detrimental to a woman's health because it depresses the function of the ovaries and instigates the hypothalamus to signal the pituitary gland in secreting luteinizing and follicle-stimulating hormones so that ovulation can occur. The use of synthetic estrogen and progesterone hormones in birth control pills also precipitate hormone imbalance. In some birth control medications, progestin is used in place of progesterone and this does not match the chemical strain of the natural progesterone that the human body produces. This is considered inorganic and harmful to the homeostasis of the female sex glands and the hormones they secrete.

The use of pesticides, herbicides, fungicides and manufactured fertilizers to control and manipulate agricultural produce has also been determined to cause xenoestrogenic anomalies in women. In a study conducted by Savitz, Whelan, and Kleckner, pesticides were found to increase fetal mortality and adversely affect pregnancy outcomes. In some cases, paternal exposure to pesticides negatively impacted conception and fetal mortality. Xenoestrogens are also found in plastic substances; Warshowsky and Oumano warned against the use of plastic containers to heat food in the microwave because they release the toxic chemical, dioxin, into the food. The authors also warned against drinking water from plastic bottles or containers that have been exposed to heat for the same reason. Xenoestrogens compete with natural estrogens for the receptor cells; researchers explained that when xenoestrogens are occupying the natural estrogen receptor cells in the body, the body is unable to metabolize or use these foreign compounds and an imbalance can occur.

Poor nutrition and emotional imbalance have also been linked to hormone imbalance. Physicians Committee for Responsible Medicine opined that poor nutrition and emotional imbalance adversely impact the body's normal flow and functionality and as a result can contribute or cause hormone imbalance. Poor nutrition and emotional imbalance can impact other hormones secretions, functions and regulation just as it can impact the sex hormones.

When this occurs, the thyroid, parathyroid, adrenal glands, pancreas, and gonads can malfunction. Serotonin, gamma alpha-butyric acid (GABA), acetylcholine, norepinephrine, epinephrine, dopamine and other neurotransmitters play important roles in the modulation of the various body functions and are influenced by nutrition. The human body derives its nutrients from foods. I advocate eating foods as nature intended, that is, unprocessed and fresh, for optimum health. Consumption of processed foods can lead to poor nutrition because of the loss of nutrients that occur when foods are processed. A constant state of emotional stress negatively influences the adrenal glands and the secretion of cortisol. This can cause or increase hormone imbalance. Research show that improper nutrition influence hormone imbalance because the body is deprived of the nutrients it needs to effectively function.

Hormone imbalance can result in one or more reproductive ailment. Uterine fibroids (which I experienced), polycystic ovary syndrome, cervical dysplasia, endometriosis, premenstrual syndrome (which used to plague me), spontaneous abortions (which I experienced more than once), ovarian, cervical, breast, and endometrial cancers (which started to happen to me and contributed to my decision to put a kibosh on my awful lifestyle and whip myself into shape), are some health problems that can occur as a result of severe or minimal hormone imbalance. Other health problems such as diabetes, obesity, Simmond's disease, metabolic syndrome, and cardiovascular disease have been linked to hormone imbalance as well.

The link to hormone imbalance is evidenced in poor nutrition, stress, bad dietary habits, lack of exercise and general imbalanced state of health stemming from continuous unhealthy diet and lifestyle. At the basis of proper endocrine function lies what we put at the end of our proverbial forks on a daily basis. My experience shows that health and wellness is a daily, dare I say it, minute by minute, choice and decision. Morter maintained that what we eat today determines how our bodies will function tomorrow and I agree.

If your food today is sausage and eggs with buttered toast, coffee, ham and turkey sandwich (on highly processed slices of bread), high fat chocolate bar, pork rinds, French fries, baked potato with butter and sour cream and a 12 ounce rib eye steak, you will likely wake up tomorrow feeling sluggish and mentally fuzzy. If on the other hand, you ate a bowl of oatmeal with 1/2 grapefruit, apples, celery and peanut butter, 3 beans salad, vegetable smoothie, broccoli soup and sweet potato, you will likely wake up feeling refreshed, rejuvenated, mentally clear and ready for the day. The nutrients your body will use tomorrow are being consumed today through your dietary choices. With every food decision, we decide to help our cells live or die.

Let's look at how hormone imbalance can occur in a woman. My research show the normal signaling process that stimulates the secretion and release of ovarian hormones is present about every 28 days of a woman's cycle. When the ovaries are working to release an egg, a few to a few hundred follicles will mature and enlarge enough to form a cyst. The cyst is normal if one follicle releases its egg into the fallopian tube. Then the other follicles are signaled to go through the various forms and stages of reabsorption into the ovary or dissolution outside of the ovary. Sometimes, because of what researchers have identified as xenobiotic, xenoestrogen, nutritional imbalance, and other health impairing factors, a number of follicles can migrate to the surface but none will release an egg. If no egg is released, the ovaries do not make progesterone. As a result of no egg being released, the hypothalamus signals GnRH to the pituitary glands to make more follicle stimulating hormone (FSH). The increased FSH causes the ovaries to continue to make more estrogen and attempt to release an egg by stimulating the follicles to become cysts, with each cycle of stimulation, the follicles are stimulated to grow larger. The continuous stimulation and lack of egg release results in a condition called polycystic ovary syndrome. Other hormone imbalance problems such as uterine fibroids, endometriosis, endometrial hyperplasia, premenstrual syndrome, and cancers of the reproductive system to include the breasts can develop in women as well.

Overproduction of estrogen as a result of inadequate or no production of progesterone (which happens when the follicle that released an egg for fertilization becomes the progesterone producing corpus luteum) can cause bloating, oversensitivity, insomnia, moodiness, and depression to mention a few effects. One of the roles of estrogen hormone is to prepare the uterus for pregnancy; it does this by causing proliferation of the endometrial lining. Working with progesterone to control the extent of proliferation, sloughing of the endometrial lining occurs, in the form of menstruation, when there is no pregnancy. Estrogen dominance can cause over-proliferation of the endometrium thereby leading to endometrial hyperplasia, essentially endometrial cancer development, if care is not taken.

Hormone imbalance can occur from over abundance or inadequate amounts of estrogen or progesterone. A group of authors opined that imbalance of estrogen or progesterone can cause many reproductive and other anatomical problems. The role of progesterone is to balance estrogen and vice versa. Research has so far revealed that abundance of estrogen hormones in the body can cause more severe problems than those linked to over abundance of progesterone. The table on page 12 presents some of the health concerns and problems that are presently associated with the physiological effects of estrogen dominance, the role of progesterone in countering estrogenic effects, physiological effects of progesterone dominance, and the role of estrogen in countering progesterone effects. Just as it is with everything in Nature, dear Mother balances everything out. Estrogen and progesterone are hormonal yin and yang in women. These hormones also need the alkaline/acid balance, stemming from our diets, in order to work well. As you will see in the table, these hormones do more for us than help keep the human race from extinction.

Estrogen Effects	Progesterone Effects
Causes breast cell stimulation	Protects against breast fibrocysts
Creates proliferative endometrium	Maintains secretory endometrium
Increases body fat and weight gain*	Helps use fat for energy
Causes salt and fluid retention*	Acts as a natural diuretic
Causes depression, anxiety and headaches*	Acts as a natural antidepressant and calms anxiety
Causes cyclical migraines*	Prevents cyclical migraines
Causes poor sleep patterns*	Promotes normal sleep patterns
Interferes with thyroid hormone function*	Facilitates thyroid hormone function
Impairs blood sugar control*	Helps normalize blood sugar levels
Increases risk of blood clots*	Normalizes blood clotting
Has little or no libido effect*	Helps restore normal libido
Causes loss of zinc and retention of copper*	Normalizes zinc and copper levels
Reduces oxygen levels in all cells*	Restores proper cell oxygen levels
Causes endometrial cancer*	Prevents endometrial cancer
Increases risk of breast cancer*	Helps prevent breast cancer
Increases risk of prostate cancer*	Decreases risk of prostate cancer
Restrains bone loss	Stimulates new bone formation
Reduces vascular tone (dilates blood vessels)	Improves vascular tone
Triggers autoimmune diseases*	Prevents autoimmune diseases
Creates progesterone receptors	Increases sensitivity of estrogen receptors
Relieves hot flashes	Necessary for survival of embryo
Prevents vaginal dryness and mucosal atrophy	Precursor of corticosteroid biosynthesis
Increases risk of gallbladder disease	Prevents coronary artery spasm and atherosclerotic plaque
Improves memory	Causes sleepiness, depression**
Improves sleep disorders	Causes digestive problems**
Improves health of urinary tract	
Relieves night sweats	
* indicates that these effects are caused by estrogen dominance or an imbalance of estrogen caused by too much estrogen and/or too little progesterone. ** indicates that these effects are caused by an excess of progesterone.	

From this table, you are able to gather that estrogen dominance can have detrimental effects in the human body and especially in women. At the same time, its role is important to survival and general body health. Progesterone acts as the balancer and curbing agent for too much estrogen. However, dominance of progesterone in the body also has some negative health effects. As a result, it becomes important to maintain hormone balance in order to prevent dominance of one hormone over another.

Ailments and conditions that have been linked to estrogen dominance include: acceleration of the aging process, allergy symptoms, autoimmune disorders such as lupus erythematosis, thyroiditis, Sjögren's disease, breast cancer, breast tenderness, cervical dysplasia, copper excess, cold hands and feet, decreased sex drive, depression with anxiety or agitation, dry eyes, early onset of menstruation, endometrial cancer, fat gain (especially around the abdomen, hips and thighs), fatigue, fibrocystic breasts, foggy thinking, hair loss, gallbladder disease, headaches, hypoglycemia, infertility, increased blood clotting (increasing the risk of pulmonary embolism, thrombosis and stroke), irregular menstrual periods, memory loss, mood swings, premenstrual syndrome, osteoporosis, magnesium deficiency, uterine fibroids, water retention, bloating, zinc deficiency, insomnia, irritability, polycystic ovary syndrome, sluggish metabolism, premenopausal bone loss, prostate cancer (in men), and thyroid dysfunction that mimics hypothyroidism.

Wow, it sounds dire and dooming when you really start to think about it but, all is not lost. Hormone imbalance is preventable and thank goodness for dear Mother Nature, the answer is literally in returning to Her. How do we do that? How do we prevent hormone imbalance and get back to maintaining emotional balance? Modern science is showing that age old remedies are the answer. I recommend proper nutrition, daily physical exercise, emotional well being (which I will expand on in the next chapter), and control of environmental toxins. According to Barnard, inadequate proportions of the chemicals, nutrients and minerals that the body requires for effective functioning can influence chemical imbalance. I advocate the intake of foods rich in the nutrients, minerals and chemicals that the body needs as the measure for prevention and treatment. Nutrition has been identified as the central preventative measure; accompanied with physical activities, control of environmental toxins, and psychological well being, any woman can achieve effective preventative measure.

On some occasions when I have consulted with women about emotional balance, socioeconomic status was identified as a great influence in a person's ability to afford the cost associated with proper nutrition, herbal and phytonutrient supplements (as deemed necessary), and general maintenance of a healthy lifestyle.

What I did was help my clients find ways to eat healthy and live a healthier lifestyle without experiencing financial hardship. So it is possible to eat healthy on a budget.

Getting back to preventing hormone imbalance, research show that consuming foods high in saturated and trans fats impair biological functioning and cause health problems. In women, high fat diets have been associated with breast cancer and other reproductive system problems. One explanation stated that fat cells cause continuous secretion of estrogen hormones. Normal weight maintenance is therefore important to prevention of hormone imbalance. Underweight women are at risk just as overweight women; severely underweight women are likely to cease having a menstrual cycle because the body does not have enough fat cells to aid gonadal hormone secretion and production, it is strongly recommended to maintain a balance of nutritive foods that will supply adequate amounts of carbohydrates, proteins and trace fats as well as the vitamins and minerals nutrients that the body needs.

Nutrition education is very important to disease prevention. Barnard and Jensen suggest in depth knowledge of foods and the nutrients they supply in order to make an informed diet decision. Nutrition information has revealed that many foods that could be thought to not have fats in them do contain small amounts of fats; when consumed, these foods provide the body's needed fat, which is a very small amount. When foods high in fat are consumed, the body's minimal requirement is supplied as well as excess fats, which are then stored. Barnard and McDougall therefore recommend a diet from these food groups—whole grains, legumes, vegetables, fruits. These foods are rich in carbohydrates, proteins, and trace fats that will sufficiently provide what the body needs. Too much fat from vegetable sources can also become detrimental to the human body. Some vegetable fats derived from olives, avocados, coconuts, seeds and nuts are advised to be eaten sparingly because of the high contents of fats they contain. I always recommend eating whole foods instead of the processed version of the food. For examples, eat olives instead of olive oil, eat whole ground flax seeds instead of flax oil. Oils of vegetables are useful in skin care products and, get this, your body is still absorbing the fats from these skin care products. Moreover, we do not need as much fat as we are consuming and it is simply wise to cut down, even on the good fats.

McDougall and Barnard maintain that fat is fat whether from an animal or plant source and a little goes a long way in humans. These authors maintain that the body processes fats the same way; the lipoprotein lipase enzyme, which is the fat extraction and storage enzyme, extracts the fat from foods that are eaten and store them in the cells until they are needed. These authors also explain that fat is stored as eaten and is not converted to energy unless the body really does need it. Why does the body do this? Because it will need to utilize more energy to convert fat into glycogen and glucose and it will delay the process until it becomes necessary.   It is even more critical for women to watch their fat intake because a woman's body is designed to store more fat than the body of a man; this is because of the reproductive functions our bodies are designed to undertake. As a result, women have more fat receptors than men. Because of this, the potential problems that fats can cause, and estrogen's contributions to fat manufacturing and storage, it becomes important that a woman's diet is balanced with the right amounts of carbohydrates, proteins, and fats and aerobic and anaerobic physical activity that will help the body utilize the energy.

Daily exercise activities such as brisk and long walks, bicycling, swimming, power walking, weight training and sporting activities like volley ball and basket ball become important to prevention of hormone imbalance. I don't recommend jogging or running because these activities are not compatible with our biological architecture.   Let me explain further, animals designed to run have completely different anatomical and dietary needs in comparison with humans. When a person is running, there is the release of hormones that are typically released when our lives are in danger.   Constant release of fight or flight hormones stress the body and makes it think your life is in perpetual danger. More so, there is nothing holding your internal organs in place and running can jar things up leading to complicated health problems. It gets worse if you have a sizeable cleavage; multiple sports bra, worn at once, didn't make the juggling and itching any easier when I had to run while serving my country and I thoroughly hated that part of my service. The much needed aerobic exercise can be attained from activities that do not hinder our health and are natural to our physiology. A brisk walk on a treadmill or elliptical machine or outside when the weather is pleasant, a few laps in the pool, one hour on the recumbent bike, or a nice bike ride through your town, will provide the much needed aerobic conditioning your body needs. If you have a gym membership or participate in group aerobic activities, forty five minutes of cardio kickboxing, Zumba, Salsa or step aerobics will work too. Better yet, you can put on some fast beat music at home and dance to your health for one hour. Hey, I do it and it's pretty fun. It does not feel like exercise and that's why it's so cool to do it. All my brain thinks about is the fun I am having shaking my butt to songs I love to dance to and my body benefits from the movement. Try it and let me know if you become addicted to dancing as I am.

Daily exercise is very important to our wellbeing. Some bio-psychologists explained that exercise activities induce the release of endorphins and neurotransmitters that aid the healthy state of the endocrine system. Exercise also acts as a stress reliever and is therefore important for women; this is because stress has been linked to hormone imbalance. An unstressed body and mind aids proper functioning of the neurological, endocrinal, and reproductive systems. Moreover, weight training and other anaerobic exercises prompt the body to use the energy it has as well as the stored fat. Since muscles use more energy when they are exercised, it is recommended to engage in activities that will engage the muscular system. Soft muscle organs such as the heart also benefit from physical activities. The combination of exercise and diet, along with emotional balance greatly influence balance of hormones in the endocrine system. Additionally, taking measures to control exposure to xenoestrogenic and xenobiotic pollutants, inorganic chemicals, iatrogenic culprits and dioxins become important to endocrinal and emotional wellness. To attain this, I recommend purchasing and eating fresh organically grown produce, green and unprocessed foods, using stone or granite cookware that have not been coated with harmful chemicals, or using ceramic or glass ware for cooking, refraining from microwaving foods, excessive or unnecessary use of prescription and non-prescription medications, and avoiding birth control pills. Lee, Zava and Hopkins recommend using natural birth control measures, environmental and consumer awareness, and product information knowledge. I always encourage my clients to become informed about the products they are consuming externally. A non-profit organization dedicated to investigating the truth in consumer products ingredients, the Environmental Working Group, has helped me help my clients. I refer many to the organization's website where they can find the toxicity level of chemicals and the truth about the ingredients on almost all personal hygiene products. If you also want to know about organic companies and their practices, subscribe to the newsletter from Organic Consumers Association; they have helped me become more informed about agricultural practices. Becoming more aware and informed about nutrition and other important health factors that influence healthy well-being and practicing them are key to preventing hormone imbalance and maintaining emotional balance.

In the next chapter, we will explore natural remedies for hormone imbalance. Many of these remedies are available in your produce section and require daily consumption for effectiveness. Yes I am talking about your food. But I will venture further and provide herbal remedies that you can prepare yourself (simply turn to the herbal remedies section for more about this) or if you are not comfortable preparing them, you can purchase them at your supplements store. If you are purchasing packaged herbs, please follow the recommended dosages or better yet, talk to your herbalist about the right dose to take as manufacturers make these herbs in varying strengths and doses, also everyone's needs are not the same.

Treating Hormone Imbalance

There are several recommendations for treating and correcting hormone imbalance problems. From the perspective of nutrition and herbs, buy and eat foods that are not treated with pesticides, herbicides and chemical fertilizers. Eat foods rich in soluble and insoluble fiber such as whole grains, legumes, vegetables and fruit, and take whole vitamin and mineral (micronutrients) supplements from food sources as well as whole herbal supplements. It has been my experience that nutrition balance, supported with whole foods vitamins, minerals and herbal supplements, will aid the body's natural ability to correct the problems. I also strongly encourage you to begin a daily exercise regimen, and spend thirty to sixty minutes focusing on breathing, meditating and positive imagery in order to gain total body, mind, and spirit wellness.

From a naturopathic perspective, ailments and diseases are regarded as an imbalance of the body resulting from a disturbance in performance. This disturbance can be because of bad diet, emotional stress, environmental factors—pesticides, herbicides, dioxin, other chemical exposures, and lack of physical activity. Many naturopaths, naturalists, holistic health practitioners and allopathic health practitioners who believe in natural remedies have used a holistic response approach to treat and reverse hormone imbalance problems in many women.

In my practice, I use multimodal holistic approach, crafted from many areas of natural health studies I have undergone, to assist my clients. To me, a multimodal holistic approach provides the most comprehensive modalities for addressing matters negatively impacting the balance of the spirit, mind and body and it is quite effective. This approach also allows me to individualize protocols for my clients and this makes it possible to treat each client's unique situation instead of a "one size fits all" approach. In essence, I have many tools in my toolbox which allows me to work with my clients from many dimensions and increase their results.

Generally, I hear people respond that healthy living is expensive. An individual's socioeconomic status influences the ability to become and remain psychologically and physiologically balanced. Food, health care, medicine and effective physiological care have associated costs. Physicians Committee for Responsible Medicine surveyed what a person, whose socioeconomic status is poor, eats. The typical diet consists of fast food burgers, fried chicken, pizza, potato chips, and sodas. Often times, fruit and vegetable presence in these foods are in the form of the small piece of iceberg lettuce leaf, a slice of tomato, a ring of onion, some pickled cucumber pieces, and fried potatoes. This typical diet has also been found to be the staple of some people who can afford to eat healthy but do not eat as such. This committee of physicians attribute this to a lack of knowledge about the importance of proper nutrition for body functioning and repair when needed. Through a treatment approach that combines proper nutrition consisting of whole grains, legumes, vegetables and fruits, herbal and micronutrients supplements, daily exercises, emotional and spiritual balance, and control of exposure to environmental malcontents, a woman's physiological balance can be achieved and hormone imbalance can be corrected.

This treatment approach is mitigated by a person's socioeconomic wellbeing because organic foods, micronutrients and herbal supplements can be expensive. Typically organically grown foods cost about fifty cents or more when compared to the agro-chemically grown produce that is available. Recommendations that can reduce the socioeconomic burden of beginning and maintaining a healthy lifestyle include purchasing bulk organic whole grain and legumes because the cost is significantly less in comparison with packaged organic whole grains and legumes, joining a co-operative for discount purchasing, joining a community supported agriculture program for crop sharing (this reduces the cost for vegetables and can increase consumption of seasonal vegetables), purchasing fresh vegetables and fruits from farmer's markets instead of stores, taking brisk or long walks and stretches for exercise, walking more instead of driving or taking public transportation (for short distances), engaging in something emotionally and spiritually satisfying such as meditating, having a quiet time, lessening exposure to violent television shows or movies, keeping a journal of thoughts and activities, re-engaging one's religious or spiritual focus, helping others by volunteering or any other means, and making time for oneself to relax, unwind, or play.

Further, the use of herbal remedies aid nutrition, physical activities, and emotional balance in correcting hormone imbalance. Some herbal remedies that have been recognized as effective for the treatment of hormone imbalance include: black cohosh, blue cohosh, chaste berry, dong quai, milk thistle, evening primrose, borage, partridge berry (squaw vine), false unicorn root, prickly ash, chamomile, cramp bark, fenugreek, ginger, garlic, red raspberry, motherwort, lady's mantle, sarsaparilla, saw palmetto, red clover, ginseng, nettle, dandelion root, yellow dock root, artichoke, burdock root, turmeric, ashoka, musta, white oak bark, manjistha, goldenseal, witch hazel bark, and feverfew. Herbs such as black cohosh, blue cohosh, chaste berry, partridge berry, dong quai, red clover, red raspberry, false unicorn root, prickly ash, cramp bark, fenugreek, ginger, garlic, motherwort, saw palmetto, sarsaparilla, ashoka, lady's mantle, musta, white oak bark and manjistha aid the balancing of reproductive hormones and influence proper functioning of the endocrine system. Herbs such as goldenseal, yellow dock root, artichoke, dandelion root, and milk thistle cleanse the liver and work together with other herbs, nutrition and exercise to influence proper functioning of the adrenal glands and the endocrine system in general. Some of these herbs, such as those in the allium family: garlic, turmeric and ginger, manjistha; ashoka, chaste berry, burdock root, partridge berry, false unicorn root, and motherwort assist the body to arrest and reverse abnormal cell growth. Evening primrose and borage are rich in omega 3 and 9 fatty acids that are essential for prostaglandins (which are important for anti-inflammation).

Some of these herbs are used in food preparation as condiments and spices and their healing properties can be gained from consuming them in foods. To repair compromised endocrine system however, I recommend taking them in supplement form because adding them to food may not be sufficient for an impacting effect, especially when the treatment regimen is in its infancy.

I also recommend taking micronutrients compounds, not individual vitamins and minerals, to provide nutrients that may be missing from the food you are consuming. Why do I recommend supplementing your food intake? I'll tell you. Nutrients we gain from the foods we eat depend on the nutrients in the soil that grew the food. Generally, organically grown foods have more nutrients in comparison with its counterpart. Still, unless you get the report of the soil nutrients content with each purchase, determining the micronutrients gained from the food is not that easy. To keep the guessing game at bay and ensure your body is receiving everything it needs when it needs it, I recommend supplementing with micronutrients blend. I am a big fan of supplementing with whole foods and I am going to share with you what I take daily to balance my body and maintain my health. I take whole micronutrients that I make from whole spirulina, chlorella, maca, lucuma, noni, rosehips, lotus seeds, acerola, acai, and mesquite. This is my personal blend and I take a few spoonfuls a day with golden flax seeds to keep my body balanced. You can independently purchase these whole foods and take them each day or you can purchase as a blend for convenience. At the center, the various blends and therapeutic aids we have are sourced from organic, wild crafted, natural and fair trade sources because I am particular about health and wellness. I am now encouraging you to also become particular about your health and wellness.

From a micronutrients blend such as the one I take, you will get the bio-available and highly absorbable, and need I say it, much needed nutrients for hormone balance. These nutrients such as, magnesium, zinc, vitamin A, vitamin B complex, vitamin C, potassium, chromium, manganese, super oxide dismutase, and selenium are abundantly available in this blend. I do not recommend taking flax seeds oil because it is no longer a whole food supplement and it is expensive. Moreover, flax seeds oil is only viable six weeks from the day it is pressed; after that, it starts to become rancid. Seriously, for the money you would pay for the oil, you could purchase a few pounds of the whole seeds that you simply keep in the refrigerator to maintain freshness. To take golden flax seeds as a supplement, simply measure 1 tablespoonful which is 10 grams, grind it in a clean coffee grinder and sprinkle it on salads, oatmeal, or soups. If you are making a smoothie, simply add the whole flax to the blender and let it run. A tablespoonful of golden flax seeds provides your recommended daily intake of essential fatty acids. Cost wise, you will pay about $3.00 for a pound of organic golden flax seeds; it comes with 45 servings at 10 grams a serving with 4 grams extra. Since I like to do cost benefit analysis on just about everything, you will spend about $0. 06 a day on your essential fatty acids and other nutrients in comparison with spending $12.00 on a bottle of oil that is no longer fresh when you get it and does not have everything that Nature strategically placed in golden flax seeds for your health and wellness.

Aside from food, herbal and micronutrients supplements, exercises, meditation and spiritual wellness, adding alternative therapies such as acupuncture, acupressure, reflexology, magnetic therapy, far infrared, cymatherapy, reiki, emotional release therapy, shiatsu, sound therapy, myofascia release massage, hyperbaric oxygen therapy, marma therapy, ayurvedic massage, basti treatment, pancha karma, Thai yoga therapy, hypnotherapy, visceral manipulation, neurofeedback, and biofeedback are helpful and have been successfully used in the treatment of hormone imbalance. In my alternative regimen for hormone imbalance, I teach women how to make and use castor oil packs in conjunction with self administered massage and emotional release technique. This saves my clients money and gets them the results they need without having to come in for treatment every day. My therapeutic approach combines multiple modalities from my training in natural health therapies, Ayurveda, nutrition, and psychology. When I work individually with clients, I use protocols such as individualized nutritional and herbal plans, far infrared, magnetic therapy, hyperbaric oxygen therapy, aromatherapy, neurofeedback, HeartMath, marma therapy, reiki, emotional release, sound therapy, cymatherapy, acupressure, pancha karma, basti, Thai yoga therapy, Tui Na, and Ayurvedic massage. I have developed a unique reproductive and hormone balancing therapy from these treatment protocols and it serves my clients well. Since every one cannot come to my location, I was inspired to create similar regimen that does not require my physical presence with clients and that is part of what you will learn in this chapter.

In a later section, you will have food recipes you can immediately start enjoying for your emotional and hormonal health. The rest of this chapter will describe the self emotional and hormone balancing therapy and herbal recipes you can make at home yourself so you can save money while balancing your hormones and emotions.

From my studies and training in psychology, I learned about the amazing brain and heart and their roles in maintaining health and wellness. I also learned about our subconscious abilities and how our subconscious stores everything we have ever experienced, thought, and wished; get this, our subconscious also controls our lives! If you didn't already know this about your brain's abilities, get ready to experience an aspect of your powerful brain in a new way. Ever heard of hypnotherapy? Ever wonder if it will work on you? Wonder no more because hypnotherapy works on everyone. In fact, you self-hypnotize many times without realizing you are doing it. Forget what you've seen on television shows about hypnosis, you can't make someone cluck like a chicken every time someone says "uncle"! But you can awaken your subconscious memory and ask it to release negative emotions, increase your self confidence, and support your efforts in maintaining a healthy lifestyle.

Every emotion we feel leaves a negative or positive mark on our subconscious. Some of our negative emotions are stimulating in nature and others are depressing in nature. For example, sadness is a depressant, rage is a stimulant. With emotional release, you will learn to release your stimulating and depressing negative emotions one by one and replace your emotional storage with positive emotions. With this technique, you will walk yourself through your subconscious and remove your negative stimulants and depressants. The coolest thing about this technique is that you can revisit your subconscious as many times as you want, to remove negative emotions. If you feel like you still have residual negativity on your "hard drive", go back to it by simply follow this technique and erase it from your "computer." It's that easy. Before you learn this technique, I want you know that your hard drive will not accept anything that you consider morally wrong, inappropriate or dangerous, it will only accept good suggestions. So, what can you use this technique for? You can use it to remove negative emotions, reprogram yourself towards positive feelings, stop your stress and stop stress-related problems. Pretty cool huh? I think so. And you will think so too after you experience it a few times. To further recharge you, after the emotional release session, do the meditation session to completely relax your body and rejuvenate your system. Ok, if you are ready for the emotional release session, stop now and flip to the chapter on emotional release therapy to read the script and practice it. You can immediately read and practice the script for the meditation session or do it separately to relax and rejuvenate you whenever you need it. I like to do meditation at night because it helps me to really relax and fall into a deep sleep. Try it, it may help you the same way. A little tip from one of my clients, she recorded the scripts in her own voice and plays it whenever she needs to release negative emotions and rejuvenate herself; you may find this tip useful as well.

Okay, back to the natural healing techniques. Herbs have a lot of benefits for us. I periodically scan for health and wellness information from reputable sources and a short while ago, I came across an article from the Food and Drug Administration about how herbs have not been reported to cause ill-effects in people in over 30 years. This shows the safe use of herbal remedies and tells me that herbs are one of the safest measures we can take for our health. My caveat with herbal use always is, don't self prescribe herbs if you are not knowledgeable about it. Know that herbs are actually medicines from Nature and should be treated with the utmost respect. As it is with all things and beings in Nature, respect is very much needed if we want to seek Nature's help. Showing respect to others and ourselves goes a long way in helping us start to heal. I encourage all my clients to respect everything and everyone around them and that always include animate and inanimate objects. When it comes to herbs and food, I always recommend people purchase from sources that harvest the plants respectfully. Sustainable harvesting is not a fad; it is the right thing to do to promote our health and that of our planet. Since we all share and borrow energy from the Universe, respecting Earth and harvesting sustainably afford us herbs and food that willingly want to nourish us and keep us healthy. Plants are alive and they have personalities too! And I think, just as it is with people, they can become quite temperamental when someone mistreats them. So enough of my preaching about caring for the environment, and on to some of Nature's best remedies for endocrinal ailments. I also provide web addresses of highly reputable sources from which you can purchase the herbs you need. Please follow the measurements provided here. If you are not comfortable preparing the herbs yourself, you may find compounds of them at your health food store or online. But I cannot vouch for the effectiveness of these compounds. Another reason I highly recommend preparing your own or having an herbalist prepare them for you, stems from the kind of energy and intention that is accompanying the preparation. When you make it yourself and you know you are preparing the remedy for your healing, the healing intention, your healing intention is accompanying the remedy. Intentional preparation is so much better than the remedy prepared for mass sales. Next to making it yourself, a remedy prepared for you by an herbalist is great, because the herbalist is working with you to manifest your health intentions. Lastly, if you are not able to make it, or do not have an herbalist who can make it for you, purchase from reputable companies with healthful intentions (see some in resources). The next few pages will expand on the health benefits of herbs for women and their benefits as remedies for popular problems.

Herb (Scientific Name)	Benefits	Comments/Cautions
Alfalfa (Medicago sativa)	it alkalizes and detoxifies the body. it balances hormones, blood sugar and promotes proper function of the pituitary gland.	Enjoy as fresh sprouts for maximum benefit. Add this to salads, sandwiches, or enjoy as a snack by itself. Rinse well before eating. Organically grown sprouts are better.
Annatto (Bixa orellana)	helps reduce blood sugar levels and supports weight loss	
Ashwagandha (Withania somnifera)	helps with stress management and stimulates immune functions	increases physical endurance and energizes the nervous system, be cautious with taking this at night.
Astragalus (Astragalus membranaceus)	good tonic for the immune system. supports metabolism, combats fatigue, boosts adrenal gland function, supports healing of the endocrine system	
Bilberry (Vaccinium myrtillus)	helps control insulin levels, helpful in managing stress and anxiety	not for those with diabetes unless taken under supervision of a knowledgeable health professional
Blessed Thistle (Cnicus benedictus)	supportive herb in reversing myriad of female disorders; provides healing support for the liver thereby helping the body eliminate toxins	if harvesting your own, handle with care to avoid skin irritation
Burdock (Arctium lappa)	good blood purifier. helps restore proper liver and gallbladder function; relieves menopausal symptoms	interferes with iron absorption, must be taken with caution

Herb (Scientific Name)	Benefits	Comments/Cautions
Calendula (Calendula officinalis)	helps regulate the menstrual cycle and reduces inflammation	
Chamomile (Matricaria recutita or Matricaria chamomilla)	Useful for reducing menstrual cramps; good for relieving stress and anxiety	
Chaste Tree (Vitex agnus castus)	general tonic for the female reproductive system; relieves cramps; regulates and normalizes menstrual cycles and hormone levels; good in relieving symptoms of menopause and PMS	also known as chaste berry. not to be used during pregnancy
Chuchuhuasi (Maytenus krukovit)	supports adrenal gland and regulates menstrual cycles	traditionally used in the rainforest as a stimulant for sexual desire
Cinnamon (Cinnamomum verum)	warming and supports metabolism of fats; helps reduce uterine hemorrhaging	not to be used in large quantities during pregnancy
Corn silk (Zea mays)	relieves premenstrual syndrome, reduces edema, helps keep the urinary tract clean	this is the tassel of the common corn/maize that we eat.
Cramp Bark (Viburnum opulus)	relieves menstrual cramps, pain, and muscle spasms	not to be used during pregnancy
Dandelion (Taraxacum officinale)	blood cleanser, relieves menopausal symptoms, liver aid	this pesky weed is good for the body; if you are picking the ones growing on your lawn, don't use harmful chemicals and fertilizers on your lawn. not to be combined with prescription diuretics. not recommended for those suffering from gallstones or biliary tract obstruction

Herb (Scientific Name)	Benefits	Comments/Cautions
Devil's Claw (Harpagophytum procumbens)	good for pain, inflammation and menopausal symptoms	do not use during pregnancy
Donq quai (Angelica sinensis)	antispasmodic, pain reliever, strengthens the reproductive system; improves the blood; helps the body to effectively use hormones; helpful in treating hot flashes, menopausal symptoms, vaginal dryness, and premenstrual syndrome.	do not use during pregnancy, if diabetic or sensitive to light
False Unicorn Root (Chamaeliruim luteum)	balances female reproductive system, helpful in treating infertility, premenstrual syndrome, menstrual irregularities. Also a good aid in preventing miscarriage	also known as Helonias. This herb is worth the money. An interesting note, part of its botanical name, "luteum" tells you something about how it influences luteinizing hormone and the corpus luteum; a perfect aid for the ovaries
Golden Flax Seeds (Linum usitatissimum)	promotes healthy skin, strong bones, nails and teeth. Aids is correcting female disorders and inflammation	also a great source of soluble and insoluble fiber; excellent source of essential fatty acids
Ginger (Zingiber officinale)	warming for the body, reduces cramps, inflammation and cramps. good in reducing hot flashes	large quantities can upset the stomach
Ginseng (Panax quinquefolius)	strengthens the reproductive and adrenal glands; supports treatment for infertility, stress, fatigue	not for pregnant women, those with hypoglycemia or women who are nursing
Goldenseal (Hydrastis canadensis)	cleansing for the body; regulates menses, reducing uterine bleeding; strengthens the immune system; fights inflammation and infection	not to be used for prolonged periods, not to be used when pregnant

Herb (Scientific Name)	Benefits	Comments/Cautions
Gotu Kola (Centella asiatica)	supports elimination of excess fluids; boosts sex drive	this herb is a good brain tonic. I use it for endocrine balance as a supporting herb for the pineal and pituitary glands
Hawthorn (Crataegus laevigata)	supports reduction of fat deposit levels, fights anemia	generally used as a heart tonic, this herb is also good for immunity
Lady's Mantle (Achillea millefolium)	helpful in regulating menstruation, eases cramping and reduces excessive bleeding. Good to steep and douche for relieving vaginal irritation	do not use during pregnancy; not for those who are sensitive to the sun
Maca (Lepidium meyenii)	relieves menstrual problems, supports normal function of the endocrine system, boosts energy, fights chronic fatigue syndrome, relieves anemia, supports menopausal transition	this root is an adaptogen and it is an all round beneficial herb for women
Macela (Achyrocline satureoides)	good for treating menstrual problems and menopausal symptoms	also good for overall immune support
Milk Thistle (Silybum marianum)	protects the liver, helps eliminate free radicals; protects the kidneys, stimulates production of new liver cells	recommended to support elimination of toxins that could be negatively impacting the endocrine system
Motherwort (Leonorus cardiaca)	good support of the endocrine system, helpful in modulating menstrual disorders, menopausal symptoms	not for use during pregnancy because it can stimulate uterine contractions; also tonifies the heart

Herb (Scientific Name)	Benefits	Comments/Cautions
Muira Puama (Ptychopetalum olacoides)	Balances sex hormones, supports relief from menstrual problems and menopausal symptoms	This herb is only beneficial if the form of extraction is alcohol-based, it is not water soluble nor can it be absorbed in the digestive process
Mustard (Brassica nigra)	Aids in metabolizing fat and improves digestion	I added this for those seeking ways to manage their weight. Mustard is also good for joint pain, chest congestion and inflammation when applied externally
Nettle (Urtica dioica)	Good tonic for the pelvic region; also helpful in preventing hair loss stemming from hormone imbalance	I have used this as a part of my blend to promote healthier transition into menopause and in managing anemia naturally
Oregon Grape (Mahonia aquifolia)	Acts as a blood purifier, liver cleanser, laxative; good for acne and other skin conditions	I added this for those suffering from hormone-related acne
Parsley (Petroselinum crispum)	Helps prevent multiplication of tumor cells; promotes thyroid function	This is one of the herbs I use to support healthy reproductive system. I personally juice it and take it as a shot, bottoms up!
Passionflower (Passiflora incarnata)	Gentle sedative that helps reduce anxiety, insomnia and stress	Added for situations where hormone imbalance is causing sleeplessness and anxiety

Herb (Scientific Name)	Benefits	Comments/Cautions
Pau d'arco (Tabebuia heptaphylla)	Cleanses the blood, assists the body in fighting bacterial and viral infections, candidiasis; supportive in tumor reducing protocols, boosts immunity	Added for situations where cysts and tumors are present. I also use this as part of the protocol to arrest and reverse growth of benign and aberrant cells. Don't get sucked into buying an extract or its active ingredient, it only works as a whole herb; I say this is "Big Mama's one up on Us" because scientists think they can just use the active ingredient to treat a problem and patent it to make a lot of money.
Primrose (Oenothera biennis)	Promotes natural estrogen; helps in managing hot flashes, menstrual cramps and heavy bleeding	Also known as evening primrose
Puncture vine (Tribulus terrestris)	Eases menopausal symptoms, stimulates the production of and balance of sex hormones, improves sex drive, enhances the immune system; has anti-fungal, antibacterial, anti-inflammatory benefits; general tonic for the liver, kidneys and urinary tract	I use this as part of my fertility boost herbs for both male and female clients; also to boost stamina, endurance and muscles development in athletic and sporty male clients.
Red Clover (Trifolium pretense)	Blood purifier, antispasmodic, immune booster	Good for the liver and as a general body tonic
Red Raspberry (Rubus idaeus)	Relaxes uterine spasms, reduces menstrual bleeding, strengthens uterine walls; good for managing hot flashes, menstrual cramps and morning sickness; heals canker sores	A major aid in promoting fertility in women and in managing morning sickness when taken in combination with peppermint

Herb (Scientific Name)	Benefits	Comments/Cautions
Rosemary (Rosmarinus officinalis)	Anti fungal, anti bacterial, anti inflammatory; promotes circulation, relaxes the stomach and supports digestion, improves circulation to the brain, detoxifies the liver; anti cancer, anti tumor; good for menstrual cramps	One of my best herbs for many other health concerns aside from those listed
Sage (Salvia officinalis)	Reduces hot flashes and other symptoms of estrogen deficiency; good in managing hormone levels after a hysterectomy or when in menopause	Also great as a hair rinse to promote hair growth and shine
St. John's Wort (Hypericum perforatum)	Helps control stress and reduce anxiety	Added for situations where high stress and anxiety is contributing to hormone imbalance
Sarsaparilla (Smilax species)	Hormone regulator, beneficial for infertility, and PMS	Also beneficial in treating frigidity
Skullcap (Scutellaria laterfolia)	Improves circulation, relieves spasms, cramps, and stress. Good for treating fatigue and anxiety	Promotes sleep as well
Squawvine (Mitchella repens)	Promotes decongestion in the pelvic region, reduces menstrual cramps	Also known as partridgeberry
Suma (Pfaffia paniculata)	Fights stress, fatigue, anemia, menopausal symptoms and weak immune system	Also good in naturally managing Epstein-Barr virus
Valerian (Valeriana officinalis)	Sedative, reduces anxiety, fatigue, insomnia, menstrual cramps, stress, muscle cramps	Smells like a rotten sock; best taken in a water soluble form such as tea, or in capsule form; not good with alcohol

Herb (Scientific Name)	Benefits	Comments/Cautions
Vervain (Verbena officinalis)	Reduces tension and stress; promotes menstruation	Not to be used when pregnant; best for those not having regular menstrual cycles
White Willow (Salix alba)	Pain reliever, good for menstrual cramps	Original source of aspirin
Wild Oregano (Origanum vulgare)	Good for menstrual irregularities and urinary tract disorders	Other oregano species does not have the herbal benefits of wild oregano, be careful when purchasing
Wild yam (Dioscorea villosa)	Has progesterone-like compounds, promotes healing of female disorders, reduces inflammation, muscle cramps; good for PMS and menopausal symptoms	

I hope you are not feeling inundated with information at this point. I provided the tables above to give you an introduction to beneficial herbs for women's care. The list is not exhaustive; there are other herbs that are used in treating problems plaguing women. From an Ayurvedic perspective, each client is individually treated and the herbal remedy is specially formulated for that client. That is what I do when I work one-on-one with my clients.

In this book, you are receiving a general approach to your care. It does not mean that you are not going to benefit, it simply means that the recommendations are general to herbs that will promote healing of certain disorders we face as women. Next are some remedies for the entire endocrine system, liver and immune system. When using these remedies, it is advised you only take them for no longer than six months at a time, stop for one month and then resume taking them. Generally, symptoms abate and when combined with food and other natural healing modalities, the need for constant herbal remedies subsides and food becomes the medicine we need daily. For those who want additional boost, whole foods supplements added to daily healthy food intake is recommended.

Here we go, time to return to the days when our mothers stood over the big pot on the stove and brewed up a potent herbal remedy to combat a health problem!

Remedy	Herbs**	Preparation	Use	Benefits
Be Balanced Tonic	1 part* St. John's Wort 1 part Passionflower 1 part Chaste Berry Powder 1 part Angelica root powder 1 part Ashwaghanda powder ½ part Gotu Kola powder ¼ part Ginger root 1/8 part cumin seeds	Bring 6 parts water to a boil with Ginger root and cumin seeds. While water is boiling, add powders, St. John's Wort and Passionflower into a large glass jar; pour boiled water along with Ginger and Cumin seeds in the glass jar. Cover and let steep overnight.	Drink 1/8 part twice a day in between meals.	Helps the endocrine system to find its balance. Supports all the glands and encourages proper function.
Liver Alive Tonic	1 part milk thistle seeds 1 part dandelion root ½ part Oregon grape ½ part schisandra	In 6 parts water, cook milk thistle seeds and dandelion root for 12 hours (better to do this in a crock pot).	Drink 1/8 part once a day	Supports proper function of the liver. Assists in purifying the blood and eliminating toxins from the body. Promotes

	berries powder ½ part blessed thistle	Add the rest of the herbs and let it cook on low for 1 hour. Strain after 13 hours and decant in a glass jar.		repair of the liver cells.
Immune Tonic	1 part Ashwaghanda 1 part Astragalus 1 part elderberries 1 part ginseng 1 part white willow 1 part garlic 2 parts Pau d'arco	Add all ingredients to a large crock pot, pour 10 parts water over and slow cook everything for 24 hours. Decant in a glass jar.	Drink 1/8 part every morning.	Support proper function of the immune system. Assists the body in its own natural defense against diseases.

*Part is used to indicate a unit of measure. Unit of measure could be a tablespoon, ½ cup or ¼ cup, depending on the amount you want to make at once. I do not recommend preparing more than you would drink in two days to avoid from having to re-heat the herbs and decrease their potency.

**Recommended herbs are organic or wildcrafted.

Food Facts and Recipes

When it comes to food, here is my recommendation, eat foods high in phytochemicals, increase the consumption of raw produce, avoid foods that contain additives and artificial ingredients, refrain from overcooking your foods, and learn what to eat versus what not to eat. Avoiding packaged and preserved foods can virtually eliminate eating preservatives and additives in foods. Anyone who eats a lot of processed foods is consuming a significant amount of additives and preservatives; Balch adds that the amount is at least 5 pounds a year. When sugar substitutes are added to the additive list, the consumption can climb as high as 135 pounds a year because sugar substitutes are the number one additive in the United States. I also recommend being careful with eating at restaurants that cook meals with monosodium glutamate because it has been shown to cause problems such as diarrhea, headaches, memory loss, confusion and seizures.

The consumption of raw produce decreases the loss of nutrients that can occur when foods are overcooked. Warshowsky and Oumano recommend eating plenty of vegetables in their raw state and slightly cooking them if necessary. Balch recommended eating fruits and vegetables that are at the peak of ripeness because they contain the most nutrients than foods that are under ripe, overripe or stored. I promote eating your fruits and vegetables in their entireties (except for the obviously inedible skins of fruits such as pineapple, cantaloupe etc) because most parts of fruits and vegetables contain valuable nutrients. In the case of citrus fruits, I recommend peeling the rind but eating the white part inside the skin for its vitamin C and bioflavonoid content.

Foods rich in phytochemicals have been shown to be disease resistant. They also have abnormal cell fighting properties because of their antioxidants contents. Phytochemically rich foods include cruciferous vegetables, tomatoes, citrus fruits, whole soybeans, kidney beans, chick peas, lentils and other legumes, whole grains, and other fruits. These foods are also low in fat and dense with the nutrients the body needs for effective and optimal functioning. Some of these foods also maintain their phytochemical composition after they are cooked; whole grains and legumes are in this category.

Overcooking meals can deplete the food of its nutrients. More importantly, when certain foods are overcooked, their organic structure changes and they can produce carcinogens. Meats and fish are in this category; researchers have found that fat dripping onto an open flame forms carcinogenic polycyclic aromatic hydrocarbons;. and cooking meat at high heat causes the breakdown of the amino acids and other chemicals in the muscle of the meat or fish being cooked thereby causing heterocyclic amines, another carcinogen.

As a result of this development, Barnard, McDougall, and Physicians Committee for Responsible Medicine recommend that women should adopt a strict vegetarian diet and avoid meats, fish, eggs and dairy products. The recommendation to refrain from eating eggs is because of the dense amount of protein and cholesterol as well as the indirect intake of the drugs that the chicken has been given. McDougall, and Barnard maintain that there are enough protein derived from eating whole grains, legumes, fruits and vegetables and we do not need the ones derived from meat, fish, dairy, and eggs. Too much protein creates high acidic levels in the body thereby making the kidneys and liver work harder to alkalinize the body by extracting calcium and sodium from the bones; this can in turn make bones brittle and porous.

In studies conducted by Physicians Committee for Responsible Medicine, strict vegetarian diets that comprise of whole grains, legumes, fruits and vegetables have successfully reversed health problems such as heart diseases, cancers of the ovaries, uterus, cervix and breast, fibrocystic breasts, endometriosis, uterine fibroids, leukemia, lupus, premenstrual syndrome, diabetes, and polycystic ovary syndrome to mention a few. Testimonials and evidentiary reports compiled by McDougall from his patients support the success of this lifestyle. A diet comprising these foods as well as daily exercises, emotional balancing activities, reduced stress environment, and avoidance of toxins from foods, utensils, and cookware can reverse hormone imbalance and work to balance the endocrine system.

I took these authors and others up on their claims and I reversed my health issues. I immediately began to experience relief and it is because of research and authors such as those mentioned in this book that I am now able to work with others to reverse their health problems. I have used strictly plant-based, mostly raw foods to help women reverse uterine fibroids, metabolic syndrome, cancerous cells, cysts, and prolapsed uterus. My personal story is inspiring and I am still on the path. Not only did I find a new lease on life, my spiritual life has deepened immensely as a result. With everything you are reading here, you should no longer be skeptical, but if you are, I strongly encourage you to give it a try and experience it yourself. My experience with clients has been that some issues that were not considered dangerous to life even were reversed along with all the debilitating conditions they were experiencing. I love the idea of safeguarding my body and feeling good so I can live life to the fullest. I personally do not recommend consumption of alcoholic beverages for spiritual reasons but many ask me about drinking the occasional beer or wine. My response is, keep it minimal and observe how your body is responding to the alcohol. If you feel awful afterwards, it may be better to leave it alone. With my personality, I have absolutely no need for alcohol to make a big fool of myself. I think I do really well at embarrassing myself when I am not imbibing alcohol, just ask my friends who have to apologize for me sometimes. Biologically, alcohol depresses the liver's functionality; our goal is to keep the body working properly to remove toxic substances, if the liver is not able to do its job of housecleaning because it is drunk, we are simply holding on to toxic substances that are harmful to our bodies. So, I don't recommend it, but if you must, drink a few sips of wine or sake and not the whole bottle.

Alright, let's get cooking, but first, some information about procuring best fresh foods your money can buy.

Food Facts

Let's begin the recipe section with some knowledge about shopping for food. Our food markets are flooded with packaged foods and many people do not know what a kohlrabi looks like if they saw it in the produce section. I used to make the assumption that everyone knew what I spoke about when I teach about food and after a few incorrect assumptions, I now know I need to do a little more education about food shopping so here we go!

First of all, I highly encourage you to shop the outer aisles of your food market when you are there. Best of all, join a community supported agriculture (CSA) club, a local food cooperative, or troll farmer's markets for fresh picks. The beauty of farmer's markets, food cooperatives, and CSAs is in the bite. The veggies and fruits are freshly harvested and brought to you, you are supporting your local community's economy, and you are being green by reducing your carbon foot print. Oh another thing, the produce is usually cheaper, at least they are cheaper through my CSA, food cooperative, and farmer's markets. If you have a small patch where you can grow some veggies, spend a few hours each week grooming your green thumb for your health and your vitality. You will be surprised at how many heads of cabbage you can get from a square garden. I have tiny holes, raised beds, half wine barrels and concrete grounds and I still manage to grow quite a bit of produce for us to eat. I am even bold enough to grow apple, pear, plum and apricot in wine barrels; I have not harvested any fruit yet though because the birds are eating them all! At some time in the future, I am planning to add a lemon and orange tree to my wine barrel orchard and I am presently trying to figure out how to grow beans on my side of the fence without the stalks playing peek-a-boo into my neighbor's yard.

Okay, here's what you need to know about produce to maximize their freshness and benefits for your wallet and your palate; I shall provide tips for purchasing and storing them.

Purchasing

When purchasing your fresh produce, keep this rule in mind: buy little and buy often. Buy a little at a time so you don't waste it then return to the market for more when you need it. I know, you are thinking, "heck, who has time to keep patrolling the market for fresh vegetables?" The truth is you will save more this way because you are preventing waste. You are also only buying what you need when you need it thus, reducing the overwhelming feeling that can happen when you are faced with bundles of vegetables and you don't know how to prepare them or if they will keep until you are ready to eat them. Besides, the fresher the better and you can avoid a science project in your refrigerator. Believe me, I have found a few surprises in my refrigerator in the past and some of them were scary. I still get the scary flashback twitches when I think about it; yep, just twitched.

Remember to buy in season, that's why CSAs and Farmer's markets are awesome. Also, make an effort to list the ingredients of what you will be preparing so you only buy what you need. Buying fresh gives you the best flavor, short storage time and it makes food economics sense. One rule of thumb with determining freshness, always pick the veggies that are crisp and naturally bright. The vegetable should not look like it has seen better days or like it needs to be euthanized. It should be calling to you with its vibrant natural color and it should be standing at attention, well not literally, and ready to serve your health needs if you know what I mean. Your selections should not be sad and begging for mercy.

If your recipe calls for a vegetable that is in the "I'm so sad, please don't eat me because I won't be of any health benefit to you" category, get another vegetable to substitute in that recipe. For example, if a recipe calls for kale and the kale looks like it has been dragged through the mud, get collard instead if it's fresh. No wimpy chard, yellow-patched collard leaves, or cross-eyed mustard greens should go home with you. I frankly think it is an injustice to all concerned for those vegetables to still be on the produce shelves if they look like they have been run over by a bull dozer!

Fresh vegetables mean the nutrients are still intact especially since leafy veggies start to lose their nutritional benefits shortly after being picked; yep, I'll say it again, farmer's market, food cooperatives, and CSA, hands down and give it up for fresh veggies! Wooh hooh! You've probably gathered by now that I am not a fan of packed or bagged vegetables; they are not fresh to me. I am a fan of dirt on my veggies and I don't want to keep checking the packing date or worse, find a dead frog in the bag, eeeewwww!

When buying roots and tubers -- carrots, parsnips, turnips, beets, kohlrabi, rutabaga, potatoes, yams-- buy those that are unblemished. They should not smell musty or funky. If they fail the sniff test, set them down and tell the produce manager, "shame on you" for trying to sell them to the unbeknownst consumer. Loose root vegetables are better than washed and packaged ones. Pick your own roots and select them for the size and quality. If the root or tuber is starting to grow (sprouting or a greenish tinge or as I like to call it, become knobby), leave it alone. That vegetable is ready to recycle itself to become fruitful and multiply.

Your Brassica vegetables (broccoli, cauliflower, broccolini, cabbages, etc), should have crisp fresh leaves and no yellow tints. Pick up the cabbages and examine them for their tightness and heaviness, cabbages should be tightly packed (not in package but in the density) and heavy. Cauliflowers are supposed to be white or creamy white, not beige, tan or a lighter shade of brown; they should not have any funky colored patches. As a matter of fact, leave the ones with patches alone. Pick broccoli that is firm, full of dark green florets; do not select any broccoli that is flowering, loose-looking or yellowing.

Pick tomatoes that are ripe and firm. I recommend selecting only vine ripened tomatoes, they are the best tasting. Select ones with the deepest shade of red and in cases where the tomato is naturally a different color, such as Black Krim or Yellow Brandywine, pick the ones with the deepest natural color for that tomato. If you are not afraid of getting your hands dirty, get the seeds from reputable sources (see resources for more information) and grow different heirloom tomatoes, you will be glad you did and you probably won't want to eat store bought tomatoes again.

Select onions that have green tops and you most likely will find such onions at farmer's markets, food cooperatives, or through your CSA because onions in grocery stores are picked when their tops have shriveled; this allows for maximum growth but less nutrients. Also, select onions with smooth skins and free of damp or dark patches.

Buy fresh legumes (snap peas, green beans, broad beans, fava beans, peas, garbanzo/chick peas, snow peas, yard beans etc) that are bright green and free of wrinkles (skin). I encourage getting fresh legumes that are small and still tender because they are younger. The fresh legume should snap when broken, it should not bend. Dry legumes should not have holes or crumble when you press down. If you can, ask the seller for storing and harvesting information so you are not buying legumes that has been sitting in a silo for years. The same applies to whole grains.

Further with whole grains, I strongly recommend eating gluten free grains only. Why? I am so glad you asked. Through my work, personal experience and research, wheat, rye, barley and oats (guilty by association, if the farmer grew or stored it with wheat, rye and barley) have been linked to major health issues including arthritis, seizures, Crohn's disease, irritable bowel syndrome, fibromyalgia, auto-immune diseases and more. Every client I have steered away from these grains has experienced relief.

Asparagus should not have woody stalks or whitish stalks. If it is looking woody, don't get it. Buy the ones that are crisp and firm with the buds still tight. Celery, fennel and other stalky vegetables should also be crisp and firm with no dark patches on them. Artichokes should not have dark patches; they should have silky and compact green heads.

Salad vegetables should be fresh, very fresh. If it is looking wilted, dry, yellowing or browning, don't get it. The same goes for the ones that are packed as salad mixes. Examine the contents carefully before buying. Buy head lettuces with the roots intact if you find them, the intact roots keep them in good condition longer.

Fresh green herbs such as parsley, basil, chives, cilantro should look and smell freshly picked; no brown or yellowing leaves and they should not start to wilt.

Storing

I mentioned shopping frequently to prevent waste and keep your vegetables fresh; on the occasions when you must store your vegetables, most of them benefit from being stored in a cool, dark place. Keep them in the crisper section of your refrigerator. Don't wash them until you are ready to use them and pack them loosely in plastic bags. You can also pack them in the eco bags that are designed to extend their freshness such as Peak Fresh™ vegetable bags. Do not refrigerate tomatoes; instead, store them on your counter at room temperature. Do not keep tomatoes in plastic bags, they grow bacteria. Keep potatoes, garlic, onions (except spring onions), turnips, sweet potatoes in a cool, dry and dark place. A paper bag will work well. Store fresh herbs in glass jars; add some water to the jars. Keep dry grains and legumes in glass jars with lids, preferably ones you can see through so you don't forget they are there.

Preparing

So you've bought some fresh ingredients and now you are ready to prep and start eating. I have been at this for a few years now and I honestly have my favorites when it comes to prepping and eating. Many women shy away from the kitchen because they don't have time to prepare the meals or don't know how. Let me share some equipment which have made it easy for me to become kitchen diva, well almost. My all time favorite is the Vita Mix. This gadget is well worth the bucks you shell out to purchase it. It literally saved my life when I was starting out on my healthful journey. I went from thinking, "how do I get all of these vegetables into my body?", to consuming more than the recommended servings for my age group!

And all it took was flipping the switch on the Vita Mix. The Vita Mix company manufactures and sells many blenders but my favorites are the 5300 and 6300. I bought the 5300 and it came with a dry and wet blade. I could make my own flours, knead dough, make sauces, frozen desserts, smoothies, soups and more. In 2012, Vita Mix released the 6300 and you would have thought I won the mega million lottery! I was so elated, I immediately bought one. The 6300 comes with multi switch options for whole food smoothies, hot soups, desserts so it's designed for achieving the proper consistency and it reduces the guessing game. So if you are not a chef but are willing to discover the chef in you, get the 6300 and it will help you feel like a chef until your chef gene kicks in. With the Vita Mix, you'll make all of the smoothies, sauces, soups in this book and those in the big recipe book that comes with the Vita Mix. For our purposes, substitute the dairy in the recipes with non-dairy options and omit the meats, poultry, fish etc that may be in the Vita Mix recipe book.

If you are wondering why I am advising you to spend a few hundred on a blender, well, it's more than a blender; it's a life changing gadget. It is well worth the money you'll spend on it and the return on investment in fairly rapid. My first blender is still going strong after nine years since purchase and I have not had a single problem with it. It is made with quality parts and it gets the job done. I have tried other blenders that claim to be just as good as the Vita Mix and I returned them. They didn't make the cut with me. Moreover, with the Vita Mix, you absorb the nutrients in the foods at nearly 90 percent because they are properly masticated. You get more of the beneficial soluble and insoluble fibers from the foods and they help your body to rid itself of harmful toxins at a better rate than if you chewed the food yourself. For comparison, you will need to chew your food about 100 times before swallowing it to get close to the consistency the Vita Mix provides. Let's face it, not many of us can sit there and meditate while chewing spinach because that's near what we would need to do to be able to chew that many times! So take my advice, buy the Vita Mix blender and blend your way into health heaven!!

My next favorite gadget is a juicer that does more than juice. It is called the Green Star. It is not cheap but it is worth the money as well. With the Green Star Juicer, you are masticating the food instead of the shredding and forceful spinning option of the centrifugal juicer. When the juice is prepared through a masticating method, it reduces the rate of oxidation and preserves the nutrients longer. I also like the Green Star juicer because it has other capabilities. With it, I make soft serve fruit crèmes, mochi, veggie strands and more. It can even extrude fresh spaghetti but I have not tried that yet. I have been using my Green Star for 7 years and I have not had an issue with it. I use my Green Star to extract fresh veggie and fruit juices and I make food-cicles and water sweeteners by pouring my fresh food juices into ice trays, popsicle maker or Dixie cups then freeze them for later enjoyment. These are also beneficial for your children or the child in you who wants to drink more water but want it sweeter or colored ☺!

Okay, one more gadget and we'll get to the recipes. I have a very simple gadget called the Spiralizer and I think it is one of the ingenious inventions ever conceived and birthed. With the spiralizer, you are able to turn root vegetables and some squashes into strands, thin and fat, and you can enjoy them in a variety of ways. I love making spaghetti strands from zucchini, carrots, parsnips, kohlrabi and beets and I use them as garnish or as whole meals with freshly made sauce, straight out of the Vita Mix. With the spiralizer, you can enjoy root vegetables and squashes in a different way.

Alright, I'll admit it, I am a foodie and I love my food prep gadgets. But you don't have to be a super foodie to fall in love with the gadgets I mentioned here. They make your cooking life easier.

Okay, let's get cooking! I have provided quick smoothie recipes for nice, healthy, breakfast or snack options. I like to freeze them in popsicle or ice cube trays and I eat them for dessert or pop in water to create a healthy, fresh and natural sweet water beverage. There are fresh juices for really light snack or beverage or for the days when you feel like giving your body a break by going on a juice fast. I do this in between my full bi-annual detoxification and purification cleanse. There are also, soups, main dishes, and salads. Let's eat.

Juices

Juices are cleansing and purifying in nature. I don't recommend frequent consumption of juices unless you are fasting. When fasting, minimize your activities and don't expend any energy as this shifts your body's focus from resting and recuperating to working.

The juices here are for repairing and rejuvenating your body so your endocrine system can heal. It is possible to become hooked and addicted to juicing so don't overdo it. Like all things, too much of it can become a problem.

Cleansing BeetyC
3-4 beet roots with the leaves
2 medium carrots

Wash and run beets with leaves and carrots through juicer until all roots and leaves are juiced. Pour into a large glass and add 2 ounces of pure water to dilute. Stir and drink.
*Beet juice is very cleansing and can cause nausea and dizziness, to prevent this, I advice mixing with carrots and water to reduce the speed of cleansing.
This is good for the liver, gall bladder, kidneys; it also helps to manage menopausal symptoms, anemia and menstrual irregularities.

Apple-Carrot
3 apples
4 – 6 medium carrots

Wash apples and carrots, core apples to remove seeds. Run apple and carrot through juicer intermittently, drink immediately.
This potent juice provides carotenoids, vitamins, and minerals essential to the proper functioning of your cells.

Be My Celebration
1 bunch celery stalks, washed.
Juice and drink.
Excellent for regulating body temperature, good for the adrenals, weight loss; fights headaches and dizziness, good for digestion, natural diuretic.

Take me to the Brussels
1 lb of fresh organic Brussels Sprouts
1 lemon

Wash Brussels sprouts well. Juice it along with the whole lemon (peel the skin if not using organic lemon).

Drink immediately.

This potent juice strengthens the pancreas so it can produce insulin. It's also good for balancing the endocrine system especially in estrogen-dominant problems. I recommend it as part of a dietary approach to managing breast, uterine, endometrial, and cervical cancers. Also an excellent source of vitamin c, in fact, more than its equal portion of orange juice.

CabbyStrong
1 head of green cabbage
1 apple

Wash cabbage and apple, cut cabbage into smaller parts and core apple to remove seeds.

Juice cabbage and apple. Drink immediately. If the cabbage is too strong for you, you can dilute with some water. This juice must be consumed immediately to prevent loss of methylmethioninesulfonium chloride, a beneficial compound.

If you experience gas with this juice, it is a normal response from the cleansing action of the juice. Too much gas means too many toxins have accumulated in the intestines, so dilute it with some water.

This juice is great for the intestinal tract and has a cleansing action for the digestive system. Also has high iodine content to help regulate thyroid and support proper weight management. It is high in vitamin C, calcium, vitamin A, and Sulfur. Also helps to heal duodenal ulcers, eczema, infections, and seborrhea.

V-9
1 pack celery
1 tomato
1 cucumber
1 bunch parsley
1 lemon
1 zucchini

Wash all ingredients. Run them through the juicer into a large cup. Drink immediately.

Excellent for the skin, maintaining regular function of the nervous system and promotes proper function of the liver, kidneys, and adrenal gland.

Purple Defense
¼ whole purple cabbage
½ whole green cabbage
4 apples

Wash and cut cabbages into smaller sizes. Wash and core apples.
Run all items through juicer and drink immediately. This juice has loads of bioflavonoids, vitamins, minerals, and is excellent for cleaning the digestive tract while fueling the body with cancer-fighting properties.

Super C Me
2 bunches parsley
1 lemon
2 grape fruits

Wash parsley. Peel grapefruit and cut into sizes that will fit the juicer chute. Run all items through and drink immediately.

This is a potent juice filled with lots of vitamins and minerals to boost the body. Has a flushing effect as well.

Anti-tumor
2 cloves garlic
1 beet root
6 dandelion leaves
¼ cabbage (red or green)
1 apple
1 tbsp spirulina powder

Core apple after washing all the vegetables. Juice everything and then mix the spirulina powder in. Drink immediately.

This juice is loaded with chlorophyll to boost healthy cells and flush toxins from the body. Also has nutrients to support healthy liver and increase iron; a good remedy for anemia, low energy or sluggish digestion.

Salads

Fruity-licious
1 cup fresh berries
½ cup grapes
½ cup diced apples
1 tbsp pine nuts, ground

Add fruits to a large bowl, sprinkle ground pine nuts over and enjoy.

Spinach and Tomato
2 cups baby spinach
1 roma tomato, diced
1 tbsp shredded carrots

½ lemon, juiced
1 tbsp sesame oil
Pinch of ground black pepper

Add salad ingredients to a large bowl, mix together lemon juice, sesame oil and black pepper. Pour over salad and enjoy.

Mixed Greens
2 cups mixed greens
8 walnuts, broken into smaller pieces
¼ lemon, juiced
½ apple, diced

Add all ingredients except lemon juice to a large bowl. Pour lemon juice on salad and enjoy.

Rainbow
1/8 cup shredded green cabbage
1/8 cup shredded red cabbage
1 pear, grated
1/8 cup shredded carrot
1/8 cup raisins

Mix all ingredients together and enjoy.

Carrot Slaw
1 cup carrots, grated
4 florets broccoli
4 florets cauliflower

3 dates
2 lemons, juiced
Some water

Shred carrot, broccoli and cauliflower in a food processor (3-4 pulses). Transfer to a bowl. Clean out food processor and add lemon juice and dates, add some water, blend till smooth. Pour over veggies and mix well.

Stuffed Avocado
½ avocado
1 tbsp diced tomato
2 tbsp black or green olives, chopped nearly fine

Mix the olives and tomato together and stuff the mixture into the avocado pit hole and on top of the rest of the avocado to cover. Enjoy immediately.

Zen Cabbage
¼ green or red cabbage or both, shredded
2 tbsp olive oil
2 tbsp black sesame seeds
½ lemon, juiced
1 apple, diced or shredded

In a large bowl, add all ingredients and mix together. Serve and enjoy.

Note: Shredded apple blends well and provides a sweeter variation, diced apple is enjoyed when the fork encounters the apple and you scoop it into your mouth, or you can purposefully seek out the diced apples in the salad and play a game of hide and seek.

Pad Thai Salad
1 zucchini, stripped with a potato peeler
½ cup mixed bean sprouts
½ cup raw cashews
½ red bell pepper, sliced into strips
1 green onion, chopped
2 tbsp freshly chopped parsley
½ lemon, juiced
½ tbsp sesame oil
Pinch of Celtic salt

Toss all ingredients in a bowl and enjoy. Makes 1 large or 2 small salads.

Broccoli Slaw
6 broccoli florets
3 cauliflower florets
¼ cup shredded carrots
1 tbsp coconut milk
1/8 cup raw sunflower seeds
Pinch of ginger powder
Some water
Pinch Celtic salt

Use a food processor to shred broccoli and cauliflower with the pulse speed, add carrots and cut into smaller pieces till they appear like tiny rice clusters. Pour into a bowl.

Use a small blender to blend sunflower seeds and coconut milk and some water till a smooth, slightly thick consistency is achieved.

Mix sauce with ginger and Celtic salt. Pour over slaw mix and mix well to distribute sauce. Enjoy.

Hot Avo
1 avocado, halved
½ tomato, diced
1 tbsp chopped red onion
Pinch cayenne pepper
2 small champagne mushrooms, chopped
1 tbsp almond cream
Sprinkle of salt

Preheat oven at 350 degrees. Scoop out 2/3 avocado flesh and dice, mix with tomato, onion mushroom and pepper. Spoon into avocado shells. Bake for 15 minutes. Remove from oven and top with some almond cream and salt. Enjoy immediately.

Easy Peasy
1 cup fresh or frozen green peas
1 sprig fresh basil, chopped
¼ cup chopped tomato
1 small garlic clove, chopped
1 tbsp sesame oil
1 tbsp water

In a large pan, sauté garlic and basil in water for 2 minutes. Add peas and chopped tomato, cook for 2 to 4 minutes. Remove from heat, add sesame oil and mix. Serve immediately. Sprinkle some salt over for taste.

Ultimate Salad

2 cups baby spinach
1 red bell pepper, cut into strips
¼ cup walnuts
1 apple, cut into 8th or 16th
½ cup mixed beans sprouts
½ cup grapes, halved or quartered

Dressing: ½ cucumber
1 lemon, juiced
3 dates, pitted

Blend cucumber, lemon and dates together in a food processor and drizzle on salad.

Simply Romaintic

12- 16 romaine leaves, torn
1 firm small tomato, cut into smaller pieces
2 tbsp shredded carrots
8 cashew pieces
4 slices cucumber
1 tsp raw apple cider vinegar
1 tbsp cold pressed olive oil
Pinch black pepper
Pinch ground dill seeds

Whisk oil, vinegar, black pepper and dill together.

Place romaine, tomato, carrots, cashews and cucumber in a salad bowl, drizzle dressing over and toss gently. Enjoy.

Mango and avocado

1 mango, cubed (substitute pear if mango is not available)
½ ripe but still firm avocado, cubed
1 green onion, chopped
1 sprig fresh cilantro, chopped
1 tsp fresh lime juice
Pinch garam masala spice blend (Indian Spice Mix)

1 tbsp olive oil

Add all ingredients to a large bowl and mix/toss together. Serve and enjoy.

This is also great on crackers or bread or use as filling for wraps.

Smoothies

Green Power
2 collards
3 romaine lettuce leaves
10 pitted dates
1 apple
1 cup water
Some ice

Blend together till smooth. Pour and drink.

Purple D
¼ purple cabbage
3 pears
2 cups water
Some ice

Blend together till smooth. Pour and enjoy.

Brassica
1 collard
1 kale
1 orange
1 apple
1 cup water
Some ice

Cut and add ingredients to blender, blend well till smooth. Pour and enjoy.

Apple Carrot
3 apples
1 carrot
1 tbsp golden flax seeds
2 cups water
Some ice cubes

Cut carrot and apples into smaller pieces; add to blender along with flax seeds and water. Blend till smooth. Pour and drink.

Body Restore
2 Kale leaves
3 bananas
1 ½ cups water
Some ice

Blend ingredients together till smooth. Pour and enjoy.

Salad
½ cucumber
3 romaine lettuce leaves
1 cup red grapes
½ cup water
Some ice

Blend ingredients together till smooth. Pour and enjoy.

Body Bright
2 oranges
2 apples
2 Zucchini
1 tbsp chia seeds
2 cups water
Some ice

Blend ingredients together till smooth. Pour and enjoy.

Squash Delight
1 cup butter nut squash cubes or pieces
½ cup blueberries (frozen)
½ cup blackberries (frozen)
½ cup strawberries (frozen)
3 cups water

Add all items to blender and blend till smooth. Enjoy.

Double Berries
1 1/2 cups any berries of your choosing
3 tbsp Goji Berries
2 Collard Leaves
2 cups water
Some Ice
Pinch stevia powder

Add ingredients to blender, blend till smooth. Pour and drink.

Cool-cumber
2 cucumbers
3 apples
1 ½ cups water
Sprinkle of cinnamon powder
Some ice

Blend cucumber, apples and water together till smooth. Pour and sprinkle cinnamon on top. Enjoy.

Energy
2 cup baby spinach leaves
½ avocado
2 pears
2 cups water
Some ice

Add all items to blender, blend till smooth. Pour and drink.

Hemp Balance
1 tbsp hemp powder
2 bananas
1 orange
1 ½ cups water
Some ice

Blend all ingredients together till smooth, pour and drink.

Blackberry Goodness
1 ½ cups Blackberries
1 pear
6 romaine lettuce leaves
1 ½ cups water
Some ice

Blend all ingredients together till smooth, pour and drink.

Vita-Pear
2 pears
2 tbsp camu camu powder
2 cups water
Some ice

Blend all ingredients together till smooth. Pour and enjoy.

Creamy Peach
2 peaches
2 bananas
2 cups water

Blend together till smooth.

Say it ain't Spinach

1 cup baby spinach
1 banana
1 apple
1 ½ cups water

Blend together till smooth.

Body Balance

4 figs, fresh or dried
2 red cabbage leaves
1 green cabbage leaf
1 cucumber
1 banana
1 ½ cups water, some ice

Blend ingredients together till smooth. Pour and drink.

Spice Delight

1 tbsp coriander seeds
4 sprigs parsley
2 apples
½ banana
2 cups water

Blend all ingredients together till smooth and creamy, pour and enjoy.

Flax Balance

1 tbsp golden flax seeds
2 beet leaves
1 tbsp Maca powder
10 dates, pitted
1 apple
2 cups water, some ice

Add ingredients to blender cup, blend till smooth. Pour and enjoy.

Sunny Morning
4 tbsp raw sunflower seeds
3 bananas
3 Romaine Lettuce leaves
2 cups water

Blend ingredients together till smooth. Pour and drink.

Berries Blush
2 cups frozen berries mix (strawberries, blueberries, blackberries, raspberries)
2 tbsp spirulina
1 1/2 cups filtered water
Raw honey or Agave (optional)

Blend ingredients till smooth. Pour and drink.

Super Spinach
1 cup fresh baby spinach leaves
2 tbsp AFA flakes or powder
1 ½ cups frozen blueberries
1 cup filtered water

Blend ingredients till smooth. Pour and drink.

Super Green Power
1 tbsp spirulina powder
1 tbsp chlorella powder
1 tbsp AFA flakes/powder
2 Kale leaves
2 cups mixed berries
1 banana
1 ½ cups filtered water

Blend ingredients till smooth, pour and drink.

Dandy-Kale
5 dandelion leaves
2 kale leaves
2 pears
1 mango
1 cup papaya cubes
1 ½ cups filtered water

Blend ingredients till smooth, pour and drink.

Quinoa Boost
1/8 cup quinoa (soaked overnight in 1 cup of water)
3 bananas
1 tbsp golden flax seeds
2 cups filtered water

Blend ingredients till smooth, pour and drink.

Fiber Fiber
1 tbsp psyllium hulls
1 tbsp golden flax seeds
4 apples
2 cups papaya cubes
2 ½ cups filtered water

Blend ingredients till smooth, pour and drink (this drink is very high in fiber, drink water consistently).

1-2 Punch
1 cup pineapple cubes
2 mangos
1 tbsp chia seeds
1 ½ cups filtered water

Blend ingredients till smooth, pour and drink.

Strawberry Bluff
1 collard leaf
2 cups frozen strawberries
1 cup filtered water

Blend ingredients till smooth, pour and drink.

Orange Pottage
1 small sweet potato (wash and cut into small pieces)
1 cup cantaloupe cubes
1 medium carrot
1 ½ cups filtered water
Dash of cinnamon

Blend all ingredients, except cinnamon, together till smooth. Pour, sprinkle cinnamon over and drink.

Berry Berry Antioxidant
2 cups mix of blueberries, raspberries, blackberries, strawberries
1 Kiwi
1 mango
1 ½ cups filtered water

Blend ingredients together till smooth, pour and drink.

Main Dishes

Cauliflower casserole

½ head of cauliflowers
2 green onions, chopped
1 clove garlic, minced
½ cup almond milk
½ cup cashews, ground
1 tbsp dried parsley
Pinch cayenne powder
4 slices of gluten free bread, dried and crumbled
Pinch of Celtic salt
2 tbsp water

Preheat oven at 350 degrees

Whisk ground cashews and almond milk together in a small bowl, set aside.
Break cauliflower into smaller florets.
Sautee chopped green onions and garlic in water for a few minutes, add parsley and cayenne powder then the milk and cashew mixture, stir constantly and remove from heat after a few minutes.

In a casserole dish, add cauliflower florets and some bread crumbs, pour milk mixture over then top with the rest of the bread crumbs. Place in oven and bake for twenty minutes with a cover. Remove cover and bake for a few more minutes just till top turns golden brown, remove and serve.

Rice Pilaf

¼ cup brown rice
¼ cup black rice
½ cup frozen peas (thawed)
1 small carrot, cubed or diced
1 celery, diced
1 tbsp curry powder
2 tbsp tomato puree
2 tbsp olive oil
2 cups water

In a pot, cook rice in water until soft but not mushy, remove from any liquid left over.

Heat olive oil in another pot and add rice, stir around to slightly fry, add the rest of the liquid from the rice and all the other ingredients, stir well together and simmer for 15 to 20 minutes. Add a little more water from time to time to prevent pilaf from sticking to the pot. Remove from heat and serve.

Sweet potato and Apple casserole
1 sweet potato, cut into bite size pieces
¼ cup regular rolled oats, ground into powder
1 apple, cut into small cubes
Pinch cinnamon powder
1 tsp blackstrap molasses
½ cup apple sauce
½ cup water

Preheat oven to 350 degrees

Mix ground oats, molasses and apple sauce together well.

Pour sweet potatoes and water in a casserole dish cover and bake in the oven for 20 minutes, check periodically to ensure it does not burn. Remove and drain any remaining water.

Add apple slices and oats mix, stir well to mix. Place back in oven and bake, covered, for 20 minutes. Check and remove casserole cover, sprinkle cinnamon on top and bake for another five minutes. Serve warm.

Rice Tortilla Layers
2 brown rice tortillas
½ cup green olives, diced
½ cup tomato puree
1 zucchini, peeled
½ cup sunflower seeds
1 tbsp oregano

Pinch marjoram
Pinch dill seeds
2 tbsp olive oil
3/4 cup water
Preheat oven at 325 degrees.

Blend zucchini, sunflower seeds, and 2 tbsp water together till a thick clump forms.

In a small bowl, thin tomato puree with some water, add oregano, marjoram and olive oil and mix well.

In a round casserole dish, spread out one brown rice tortilla, spread some zucchini-sunflower mixture on it; spread some tomato sauce on it, layer with second tortilla and repeat zucchini-sunflower and tomato sauce. Bake in the oven 15 minutes, remove from heat and spread diced olives over. Pop back in the oven for 5 minutes and remove. Cut and serve.

Spinach Turnovers
1 cup baby spinach leaves
1/8 cup chopped red onion
Pinch dill seeds
Pinch black pepper
1 tsp lemon juice
2 tbsp water
4 leaves fresh parsley, chopped
½ tbsp olive oil
1 tortilla
¼ cup tomato sauce

In a pot, cook the onion, parsley, dill, pepper and spinach in water; cook over medium heat and stir frequently to keep from sticking. Stir in the lemon juice.

Preheat oven to 350 degrees

Cut tortilla in half. Wet the edges with some water and add a few tablespoons of the spinach mixture to the center of each half. Fold over each side and press the edge to seal. Place on a baking sheet, pour tomato sauce over and bake for 15 minutes. Remove and serve.

Broccoli Bake

½ cup soft tofu, mashed
½ green bell pepper, diced
½ cup cooked brown rice
1 cup broccoli
Pinch garlic powder
Pinch cayenne pepper
Pinch Celtic salt
½ cup almond milk

Preheat oven at 350 degrees. In a casserole dish, mix mashed tofu, bell pepper, rice and broccoli together with almond milk. Sprinkle garlic and cayenne powder on top and bake for 30 minutes. Remove from heat and sprinkle Celtic salt on top, serve warm.

Bean cake

½ cup black eye peas, soaked in 1 cup water for 30 minutes

1 red bell pepper
¼ small red onion
2 tbsp olive oil

Use hands to rub black eye peas and remove skins, wash with water, strain and repeat washing and straining until most of the skin is removed. Soak for another 1 hour and then transfer to a blender. Blend with some water until a thick consistency is achieved.

Preheat oven to 350 degrees.

Pour into a glass bake dish precoated with some oil. Add the bell pepper and onion and oil. Stir well to distribute. Cover and bake till firm (insert a knife and remove, bean cake is ready when knife comes out clean). Cut and enjoy. Good warm or cold.

Rice Medley
½ cup wild rice blend
2 green onions, chopped
4 button mushrooms
1 ¼ cup water
1 tbsp tomato puree
1 tsp white miso paste
½ cup frozen peas (thawed)

Bring water to a boil in a pot, add wild rice blend and bring to a boil again, reduce heat, cover and simmer for 45 minutes. Mix tomato puree and miso paste together with some water to thin out. Add peas to wild rice, add mushrooms and chopped green onion then tomato-miso sauce. Stir well with rice and let simmer further for another 15 minutes, check occasionally. Remove from heat and serve warm.

Spinach Paneer and Tortilla
1 cup baby spinach, chopped well
2 tbsp pine nuts
1 tbsp raw walnuts
1 tsp lemon juice
Pinch ginger powder
Pinch garam masala
½ tbsp minced garlic
Dash ground black pepper
1/8 red bell pepper, diced
2 leaves fresh basil, chopped
1 tsp black sesame seeds

In a large bowl, combine chopped spinach, bell pepper and basil, set aside.

In a food processor, blend all the rest of ingredients except sesame seeds. Stop and scrape down the sides as items blend to ensure a good smooth mix. When smooth, pour into a bowl and mix with spinach, bell pepper and basil, mix well. Sprinkle sesame seeds on top and let marinate or 1 to 2 hours before serving.

When ready to serve, warm 1 brown rice tortilla on the griddle and cut into smaller pieces. Use tortilla to scoop spinach paneer. Enjoy.

Zucchini Bake
1 zucchini, grated
½ cup soft tofu
¼ cup water
1 tbsp marjoram
1 tsp oregano
Pinch fennel seeds
2 tbsp chopped red onion
¼ water
¼ cup oats granola mix, ground

Blend tofu and water together till smooth.

Preheat oven to 375 degrees
In a small casserole dish, mix grated zucchini, tofu blend and spices together with half of the chopped onion and all the ground granola. Pat down and bake for 30 minutes. Sprinkle the rest of the onion and bake for another 5 minutes. Remove from oven, cut and serve.

Curry-Stuffed Peppers
2 large bell peppers
2 potatoes, peeled and cut into chunks
¼ cup chopped broccoli
Pinch curry powder
2 tbsp chopped red onion
2 tbsp chopped carrot
Pinch cumin powder
Pinch turmeric powder
1 tsp lemon juice
1 tsp white miso paste
2 tbsp water
Pinch ground black pepper

Cook potatoes until soft, drain and mash well.

Preheat oven to 350 degrees

Mix miso and water till no clumps remain. Sauté onion in some miso water for about 5 minutes, stir continuously. Add broccoli, curry powder, turmeric, cumin and cook in the rest of the miso water. Mix with mashed potatoes, add lemon juice and black pepper.

Cut the tops of the bell peppers and scoop out seeds. Stuff potato mixture into the bell peppers. Cover with bell pepper tops and bake for 20 minutes

Sauce
Pinch ginger powder
Pinch curry powder
2 tbsps tomato puree
1 small garlic, minced
Some water

In a sauce pan, combine water, tomato puree, ginger and garlic. Heat for 5 minutes or until it starts to boil, remove from heat and serve with stuffed peppers.

Quinoa Tabouli
½ cup cooked quinoa
¼ cup finely chopped parsley
1/8 red onion, finely chopped
1 garlic clove, finely chopped
½ cucumber, finely chopped
4 sprigs fresh mint, finely chopped

Dressing: ¼ cup fresh lemon juice
1/8 cup extra virgin olive oil
½ tbsp ground white pepper
Some salt to taste
Mix dressing ingredients together.

Add tabouli items to a large bowl; stir in dressing, serve chilled or at room temperature

Spinach Casserole
1 cup cooked quinoa
2 cups baby spinach, chopped
1 orange bell pepper, diced
1 cup ground pine nuts
1 cup cashews, broken into pieces
2 celery stalks, diced
1 carrot, shredded
1 tsp Celtic salt
1 tbsp marjoram
1 tbsp thyme
1 tbsp ground fennel
1 ½ cups water (for sweeter casserole, use fresh apple juice instead of water)

Preheat oven at 325 degrees.

In a large bowl add all ingredients together and mix well. Transfer into a casserole dish and pat down. Place in the oven and bake for 20 minutes. Cut and serve. Also awesome as leftover lunch or snack.

Quinoa and vegetable medley
½ cup quinoa
¾ cups water
2 collard leaves, washed and chopped
2 Brussels sprouts, washed and chopped.
1 small red radish, washed and cut into small cubes
1 tomato, diced
1 tbsp olive oil
2 tbsp diced red onion
Pinch of ginger powder
Pinch of Celtic salt
1/8 cup water

Wash quinoa in some water and drain.
Cook quinoa in ¾ cup of water for 15 minutes, turn down heat and simmer until small rings are visible around quinoa. Remove from heat.

In a wok or skillet, heat olive oil. Sauté onion for 2 minutes, add diced tomato, ginger, Brussels sprouts, collards, and radish. Stir constantly for a few minutes then add some water. Cover and let cook on low heat for ten minutes.

Serve quinoa into a bowl, pour vegetables over and sprinkle Celtic salt on top. Enjoy.

Stuffed Cabbage
2 red or green cabbage leaves
1 tomato, diced
1 avocado, mashed
¼ cup walnuts, chopped
Pinch ginger powder
Pinch black Cumin powder
2 wooden toothpicks

In a bowl, mix diced tomato, mashed avocado, chopped walnuts, ginger and black cumin together. Scoop into the two cabbage leaves, fold over and press the sides down, hold in place with two toothpicks. Preheat oven at 300 degrees and bake for 10 minutes.

Brown Rice Collard Burrito
1 large Collard green leaf, de-spined
¼ cup cooked brown rice, hot
½ very ripe avocado, mashed well with a fork
1 tbsp fresh salsa
2 tbsp sweet corn
Pinch Celtic salt

Spread the two collard leaf halves on a cutting board, layer each half with brown rice, mashed avocado, corn and salsa, sprinkle Celtic salt and fold top ends in then roll from one side to the other. Enjoy.

Millet and Steamed Vegetables

½ cup plain Millet
¾ cup water
½ cup broccoli
¼ cup green beans
¼ cup carrot slices
2 tbsp water
Pinch Garam Masala
Drizzle of olive oil

In a small pot, cook Millet in water until soft, about 30 minutes. In another pot, steam vegetables with 2 tbsp water. Cover to keep heat within and steam for five minutes. Remove from heat and pour into plate with Millet, drizzle olive oil over and sprinkle garam masala over. Enjoy.

Hummus Sandwich

½ cup chickpeas hummus
2 romaine lettuce leaves
2 slices tomato
1 ring onion
1 tbsp brown sesame seeds
2 cold whole grain gluten free pancakes

Spread hummus on one pancake, sprinkle sesame seeds then layer with tomato slices and onion, half romaine leaves and place over, cover with the other pancake. Enjoy (note, this is a great but messy sandwich).

Note: spoon may be needed to scoop hummus that is trying to escape ☺

Soups

Avo-Brocco Soup
1 avocado (peeled, cored, and diced)
1 stalk of broccoli (washed and cut into smaller pieces)
5 pitted dates
1 apple (washed, cored and sliced)
1 cup of warm filtered water

Add ingredients to a hi-powered blender and blend till smooth and creamy. Pour and serve immediately. Makes 1 hearty soup or two small soups to serve with a salad.

Minestrone
1 tsp minced garlic
2 tsp chopped onion
½ stalk celery, diced
½ carrot, diced
1 cup water
1 plum tomato, chopped
½ potato, scrubbed and chopped
Pinch parsley flakes
Pinch dried oregano
Pinch dried basil
Pinch marjoram
Pinch ground white pepper
3 tbsp tomato puree
½ zucchini, diced
½ cup cooked cannellini beans
¼ cup cooked brown rice
Sprinkle of Celtic salt

Add garlic, onion, celery, tomato puree, carrot, potato, and water to a large soup pot, let cook over medium heat for 30 minutes. Add rice, beans, zucchini and spices, reduce heat and simmer for 20 minutes. Remove heat and serve. Sprinkle some salt and enjoy.

Quick Chili
1 cup cooked pinto beans
2 small tomatoes, diced
1 small garlic clove, diced
1 tsp cayenne pepper
Pinch chili flakes
1 tsp salt
½ red bell pepper, diced
½ green bell pepper, diced
1 tsp turmeric
Pinch ground cumin
1/8 diced red onion
1 1/2 cups water

In a stew or soup pot, heat some water, add onion and garlic and quickly stir to release fragrance. Add the rest of the water and ingredients. Cover pot and cook chili for 15 minutes, turn down heat and simmer for 10 minutes. Remove from heat and serve.

Sweet Potato stew
1 sweet potato, washed and cut into small pieces
½ cup whole dry peas
1 tomato, diced
1 tsp curry powder
Pinch garlic powder
Pinch ginger powder
1 tbsp tomato puree
¼ cup sun dried tomatoes
1 ½ cups water

In a stew pot, bring whole peas to a boil in the water, let cook till just about tender. Add sweet potato, sun dried tomatoes, diced tomato, tomato puree and spices. Turn down heat and simmer for 20 minutes to allow spices and flavors to blend. Remove from heat and serve.

Red beans and black rice stew
¼ cup black rice
¼ cup red kidney beans
2 cups water

½ cup frozen whole peas
¼ cup tomato puree
1 clove garlic, minced
Pinch of ground cloves
Pinch of ground black pepper
1 celery stalk, diced
Pinch of ground ginger
1 tsp tapioca starch

Soak beans overnight. In the morning, add black rice, beans and water to crock pot. Cover and cook on low.
When beans and rice are soft, add peas, tomato puree, garlic, cloves, celery, ginger and black pepper. Use a little bit of the stew water to mix tapioca starch well to remove any lumps, pour into stew and cover. Let cook for 1 ½ to 2 hours and serve.

Three bean stew
¼ cup cooked pinto beans
1/8 cup cooked kidney beans
1/8 cooked cannellini beans
2 tomatoes, diced
1 celery, diced
½ cup frozen peas
¼ cup sweet corn
1 cup almond milk
¼ cup water
Pinch paprika powder
Pinch cumin powder
Pinch cloves powder
Pinch dill seeds powder

In a crock pot, combine beans and vegetables and seasonings with the milk and water. Cook on high setting for 1 hour. Turn off heat and serve.

Squash Bisque

1 large tomato
½ tbsp olive oil
½ cup spaghetti squash
1 clove garlic
1 sprig fresh basil or 1 tbsp dried basil leaves
2 tbsp cashews, chopped into pieces
Pinch Celtic salt
Pinch ground black pepper
¾ cup hot water

Blend all ingredients except chopped cashews till smooth. Pour into a bowl, add cashews and enjoy.

Lentils Soup

½ cup lentils
1 cup water
Pinch caraway seeds
Pinch cardamom seeds
Pinch black pepper powder
¼ cup cashews
Some Celtic salt

Cook lentils in water until soft. Transfer to a blender and blend with cashews till smooth. Pour back into soup pot, add seasonings and cook on low heat for 15 minutes. Remove from heat and sprinkle some Celtic salt in the middle. Enjoy.

Tomato Soup

3 large beefsteak tomatoes,
½ cup cooked white beans
1 tsp curry powder
1 clove garlic, minced
Pinch ginger powder
¼ red onion, chopped fine
1 tbsp olive oil
2 tsp paprika powder
1 tsp salt
¼ cup water

Blend tomato, white beans and water together, pour into a small sauce pan, add the rest of the ingredients, except olive oil, and simmer on low heat for 15 minutes, remove from heat, drizzle in olive oil and serve.

Red Beans Soup
¼ cup red kidney beans
¼ red onion, chopped
1 tbsp chopped garlic
2 tbsp olive oil
3 cups water
1 tbsp paprika powder
1 tsp ground cumin

Cook beans in water till soft (use crock pot and cook overnight); add the rest of the ingredients and let cook for another 2 hours. Remove from heat and serve.

Creamy Spinach Soup
2 cups baby spinach
1/8 cup raw cashews
½ cup warm water
Pinch Celtic salt
Pinch pepper

Blend spinach with some water, pour into a bowl. Rinse blender cup and blend cashews with the rest of the water. Swirl blended spinach with cashew cream, sprinkle salt and pepper and enjoy.

Wow, all of these recipes are making me hungry. Just for convenience, I added a simple list to serve as a reminder. You can copy this list and carry it with you so you know which foods to focus on and which ones to avoid or eat sparingly.

Foods for Optimum Health	Foods to Avoid	Foods to Eat Sparingly
All leafy vegetables	Any processed food	Oils
All crucifers	Beef	4 oz salt water fish
All squashes	Pork	Whole grain wheat, Rye and Barley (except in Probiotic or grass forms)
Root vegetables	Chicken	
Seeds	Turkey	
All Spices	All dairy products	Salt
Whole grains (Millet, Amaranth, Buckwheat, Quinoa, Teff, Oats)	All other meats and meat products	Dehydrated fruits
All fruits		

Aroma Medicine Recipes

Now, let's move to another area that many are not aware of its healing effects for women, aroma medicine. Essential oils are concentrated life forms of plants and they pack a whallup of healing when used properly. Without complicating things further, I have provided some basic essential oils that I feel every woman should have in the home for her health. The oils presented here are for some general gynecology support. When applying, it is imperative you follow the instructions. Plant essences are more powerful than the plants as herbs because the potency greatly increases.

Aroma medicine is good for a variety of ailments and prevention. For our purposes, I focused on general hormones support, hormone related acne, sleep aid, premenstrual syndrome, amenorrhea, dysmenorrheal, menorrhagia, menopause, and pelvic pain. In the table on the next page, I provided simple and safe essence support for the aforementioned. There are remedies for these and other problems plaguing women but they require a knowledgeable practitioner of aroma medicine to prepare them. If you want to explore aroma medicine as an adjunct treatment approach, you can call our center and we will be happy to help you.

Here we go!

Hormone Related Acne Relief	Premenstrual Syndrome Relief
5 drops cedarwood	20 drops of clary sage
6 drops lemongrass	10 drops Geranium
10 drops clary sage	8 drops chamomile (Roman or German)
2ml distilled water	8 drops palma rosa
	2 ml jojoba oil
Mix essential oils and water together and pour into a spray bottle. Clean face very well and spritz on face; eyes closed to avoid irritation. Rub in to skin to encourage absorption. Use daily. Shake well before each use.	Mix all oils together in an amber bottle with dropper. Rub over your abdomen, hips, lower back and between the cleavage a week to a few days before your period.
Amenorrhea (loss of periods)	Dysmenorrhea (painful period)
15 drops German chamomile	15 drops sage
15 drops geranium	15 drops red thyme
10 drops yarrow	10 drops lavender
10 drops fennel	10 drops geranium

2ml jojoba oil Mix all oils together and store in a glass amber bottle. Rub the blend over abdomen, pelvic region and lower back every day for at least 2 weeks. This is a great adjunct to other protocols for correcting amenorrhea.	10 drops Roman chamomile 2 ml jojoba oil Mix all ingredients together and store in a glass amber bottle. Rub the blend over lower abdomen and lower back beginning 3 days prior to menstrual flow. Do this daily until menstrual flow subsides.
Menorrhagia (heavy bleeding) 15 drops Roman chamomile 15 drops lemon 15 drops geranium 2 tbsp jojoba oil Mix all ingredients together. Massage into lower abdomen and pelvis daily.	Menopause 15 drops clary sage 10 drops geranium 10 drops grapefruit 10 drops lemon 8 drops juniper 3 drops jasmine (must be real) 2 ml avocado oil Mix all ingredients together. Massage all over the body daily.
Pelvic Pain 15 drops geranium 10 drops lavender 10 drops peppermint 10 drops Roman chamomile 5 drops bergamot 2 drop jasmine absolute 1 drop rose absolute 2ml jojoba oil Mix all ingredients together and store in an amber bottle. Rub 3-5 drops on the pelvis and lower abdomen twice daily.	General Hormones Aid 30 drops clary sage 20 drops geranium 10 drops sage 2 drops rose absolute 2 ml jojoba oil Mix all ingredients together and store in an amber bottle. Rub in 2 drops each to your crown, behind your ears, in between your breasts and on your lower abdomen daily.

Women's Balance Essence Perfume	Sleep Well Aid
10 drops neroli	15 drops lavender
10 drops clary sage	15 drops chamomile
5 drops patchouli	
5 drops ylang ylang	
5 drops lavender	Mix all ingredients together and add 2 drops to pillow just before laying down to sleep.
2 ml avocado oil	
Mix all ingredients together and store in an amber bottle. Apply to temple, sternum, and wrists daily.	

Heart Connect Therapy

"Kindness begins in your heart. It is a seed sown by love, watered by caring, and nurtured by happiness. Be kind to your body, love it, nurture it, connect with it."

Set aside a time when you will not be disturbed. Begin by playing soft, soothing music. Light a candle and use it as your focal point.

Settle down comfortably on a cushioned chair or use a meditation cushion if you have one. Keep your gaze on the lit candle. Begin to breathe in deeply and observe the cycle of your breath as it flows in through the nose, through your lungs, down to the expansion of your rib cage, abdomen and out of your nostrils. Encourage your mind to disregard any thoughts that require processing; allow these thoughts to float in and be an observer to the thoughts. Do not process them, simply let them dance in and out as you take deep full breaths in and out.

As you maintain focus on the lit candle and breathe in deeply, begin to imagine a bright white light is surrounding your body and penetrating every cell of your body. Imagine this pure, white light energize and fill your body with deep sense of safety and security. Imagine this pure white light as a cleanser that is washing away all negative thoughts and feelings that may be keeping you from connecting with your sacred heart. Keep taking in full breaths and now with each exhalation, imagine your heart releasing all things that are holding you back. Begin to release any negative emotion or painful situation which may be keeping you from heartfelt serenity and peace. Stay in this space for a few minutes as you gently release all of these feelings into the pure white light. With each release, the pure, white light is filling the space in your sacred heart with serenity, peace, love and joy. Now imagine feeling awashed with pure love. Bask in this purity for as long as you desire.

When ready, gently shift your focus from the lit candle to the floor. Blink a few times to allow your eyes to adjust. You may journal your experience and write down any insight, feelings, ideas or thoughts experienced during this session.

Feel free to use this therapy to unfurl any issues that may become a stressful one or to even remind yourself that you are a spiritual being filled with love, compassion and harmony.

Therapeutic Bodywork

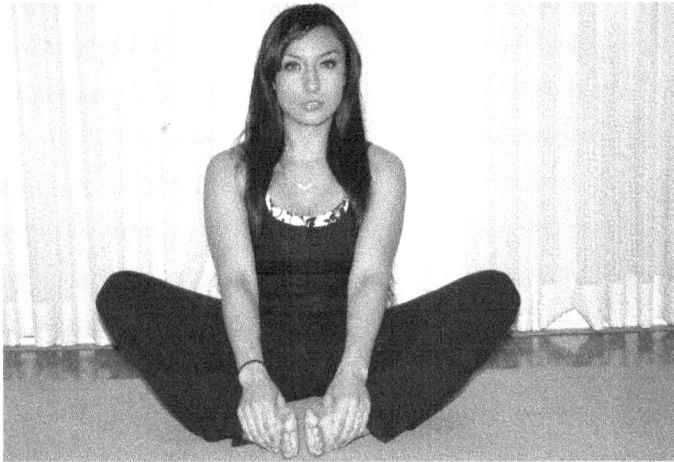

Sit comfortably on a yoga mat. Bring your feet together until they are almost touching. Place your hands over your feet with your thumbs resting comfortably on your arches. Press your thumbs down and gently slide inwards as if you are kneading dough. This stimulates energy centers located at the heart of your feet. These centers are also connected to your emotions. Gentle pressure at these centers stimulate the kidney meridian, lungs and respiratory system.

Modified view with ball of feet touching.

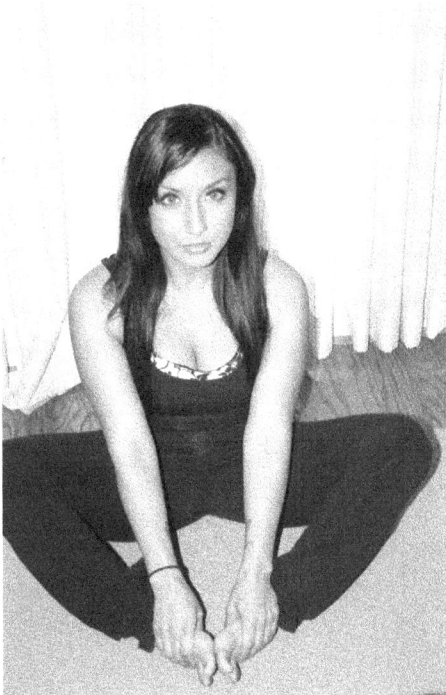

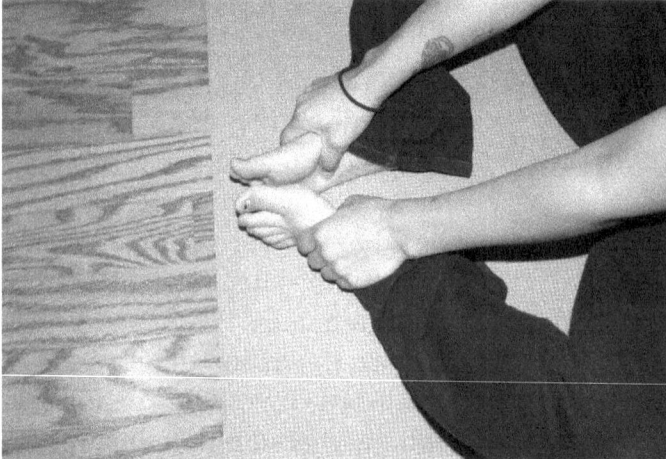

Side view

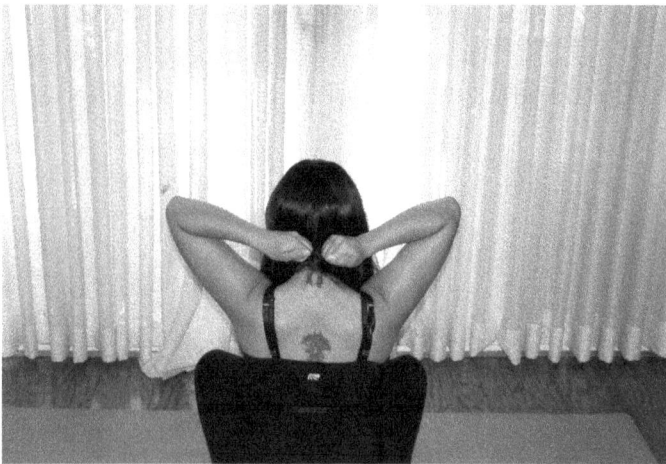

Ball your hands into a fist; place both fists, with edge of your index fingers, at the base of your skull. Gently press down, inhale and imagine water rising, exhale and imagine water falling down your neck and down to the base of your spine, at your tail bone.

This gentle pressure at the base of the skull relieves tension in the whole body. It helps to align the neck and the occiput.

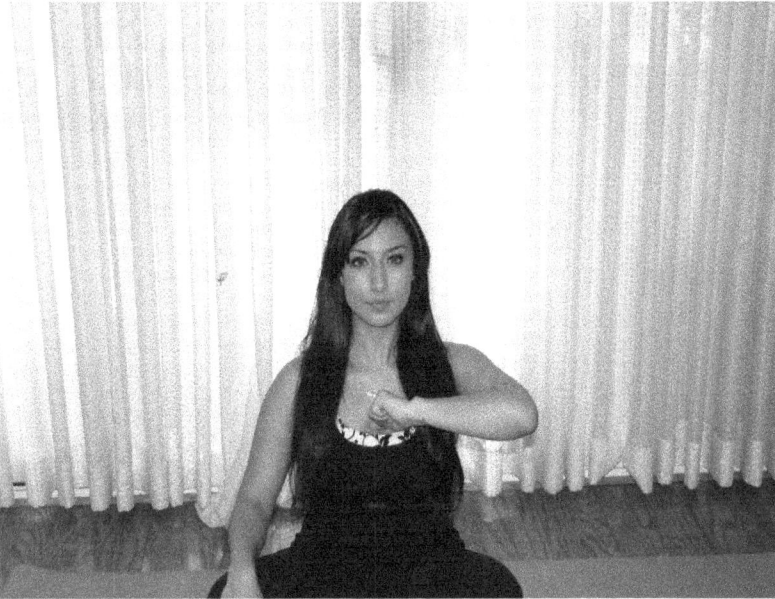

Make a fist and position the edge of your thumb directly over the heart center (the center of the breast bone). Begin a gentle circular massage in a clockwise manner. Massage for 1 minute, stop and inhale deeply into this center. Focus your breath with the intention of filling this center with divine love and serenity. Spend some time here to release any angst, negativity, or painful emotion you may be holding. As you exhale, visualize these unwanted issues leaving your being and pure love and light replacing the void they used to occupy. This center governs blood plasma, circulatory system, boosts immunity, promotes emotional wellbeing and spirituality.

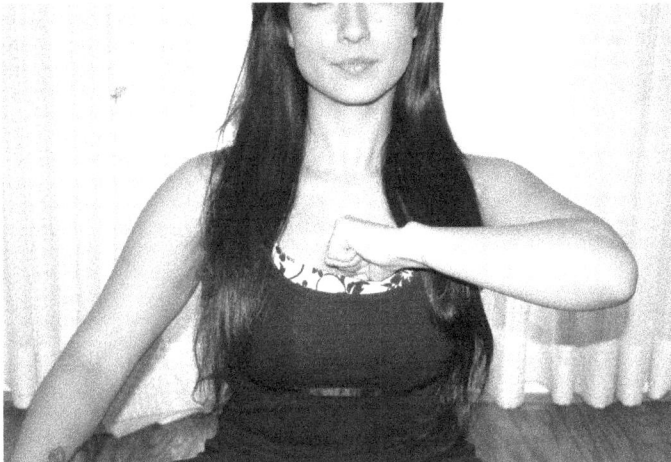

Close up view of the heart center.

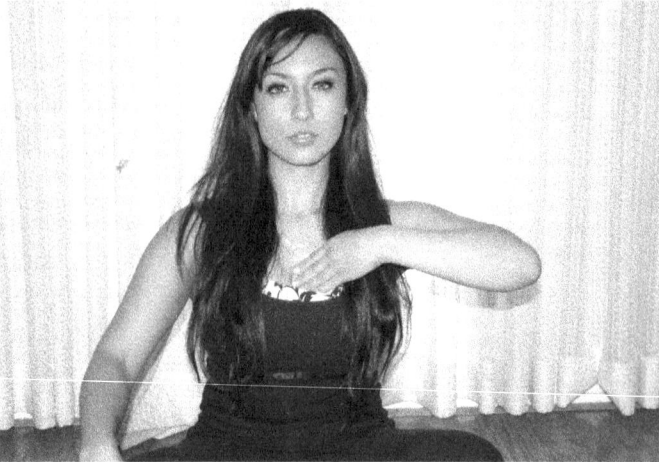

If you are unable to form a fist, simply place the tips of your finger on the heart center and complete the exercise as described above.

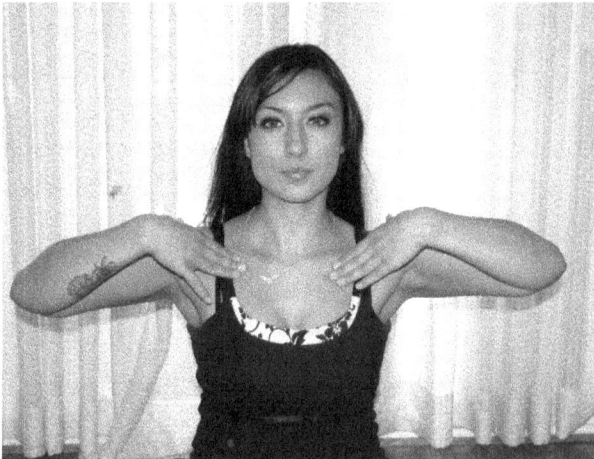

Raise your arms to shoulder height, curl in your fore arms and place your three middle fingers three inches from your armpits. Breathe in deeply and gently tap for 30 seconds. Stop tapping, breathe in fully and proceed to the next exercise.

This stimulates peripheral energy centers and syncs them with the heart center.

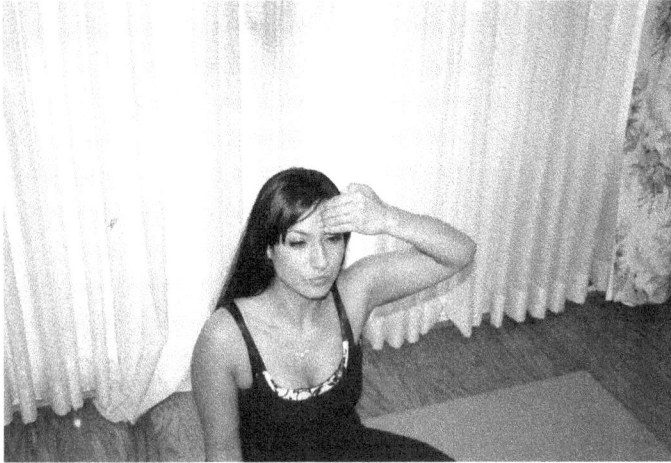

Curl your hand into a half fist; point the tips of your four fingers directly over the center of your forehead. Gently rub in a circular motion for 30 seconds to stimulate the pituitary gland. If you wish, say a prayer while doing this. I have found that praying while massaging this point helps to bring my intentions to fruition.

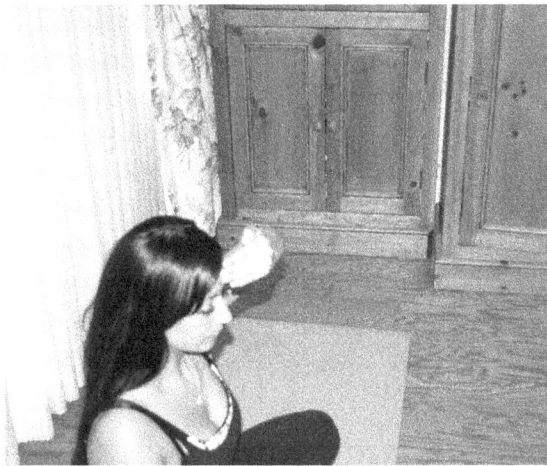

Side view

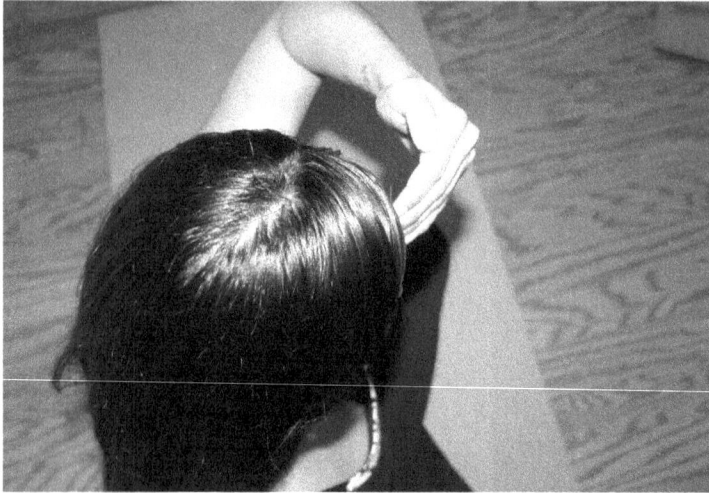

Close up view

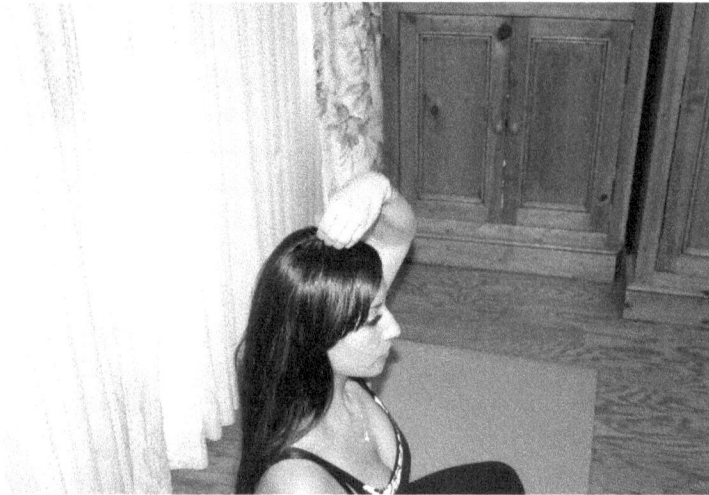

Curl your hand into a fist and place the fore part of your fingers at the crown of your head. Gently rub your crown to stimulate the pineal gland. This is an important area for general wellbeing as the pineal gland regulates many things, including our sleep/awake cycle. I call it the antenna because it syncs with the sun and moon cycles and helps us orient ourselves.

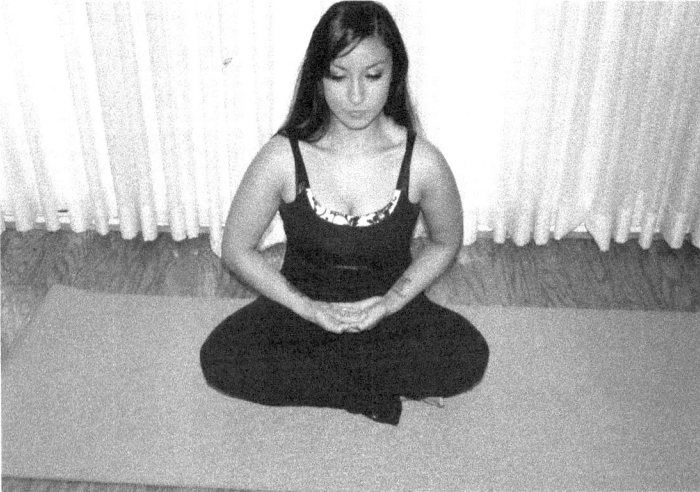

Fold your palms, right over left and connect your thumbs. Place your palms at the base of your waist (right over your pelvic floor). This area is very important to sexual energy in both men and women but more so in women. It is the seat of our emotions and it directly connects to the heart center. Make the connection with this energy center by breathing in deeply and sending your full breath to the point where your hands are resting. Imagine the breaths circling in, around the base where your hands are resting and out through the nose. This circling breath energizes this point and supports the general strength of the body.

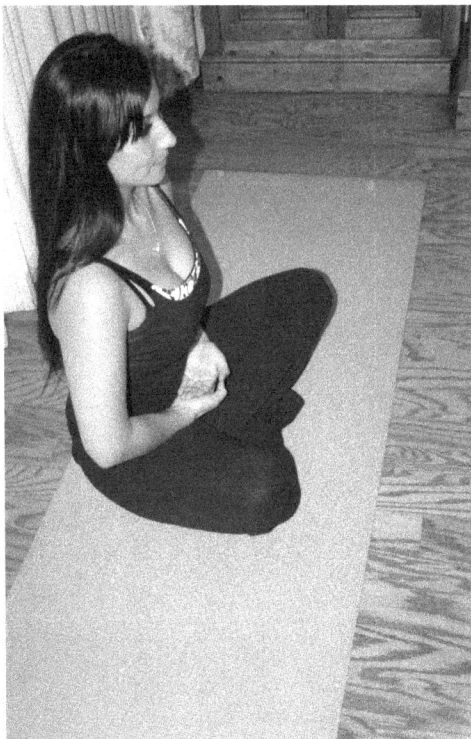

Side view

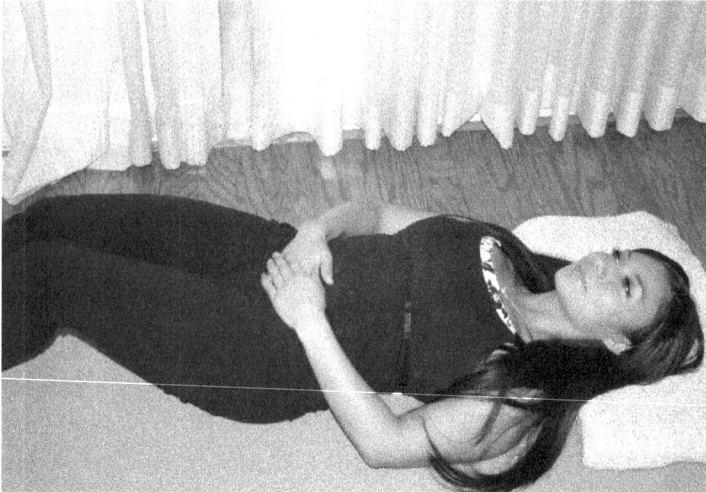

Alternatively, you can lay down and place both hands over the energy center described above and do the circling breath. Option with legs at 45° angle shown.

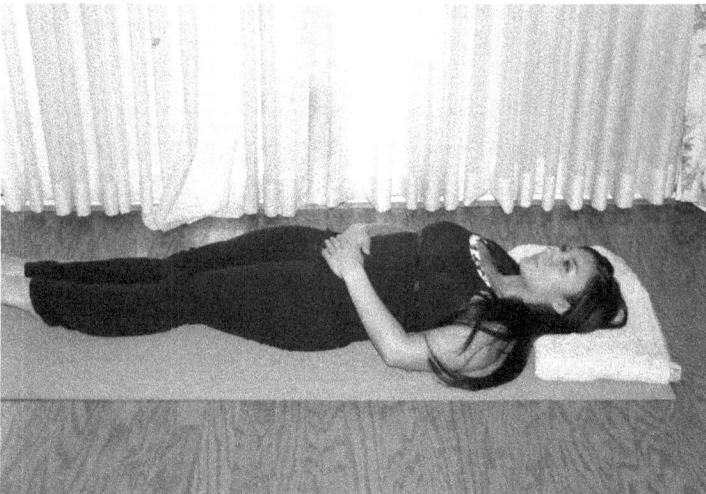

The same position as above with legs laying flat on the mat.

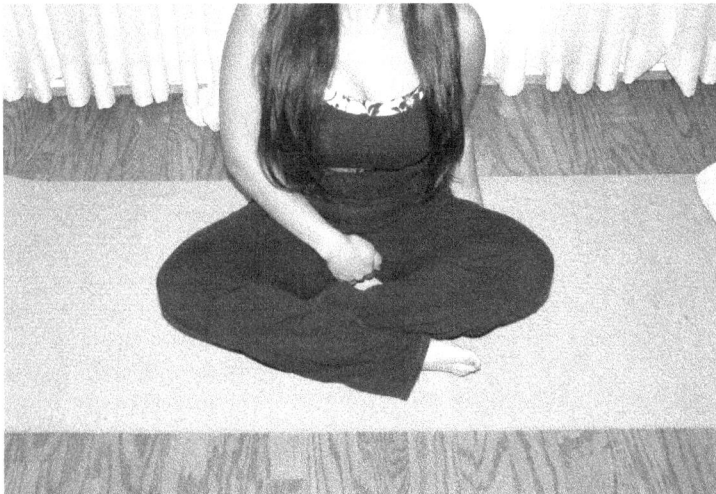

To work on this energy point, you will need to locate the perineum, which is at the junction between the vagina and the anus. Cup your hands and gently press on the perineum with the tips of your fingers. Breathe in deeply and feel your breath pulling down the front of your body to the perineum and circling back up through your spine, forehead and exiting out the nostrils. This is a powerful breath work so only do it about three times until you feel you can increase the number of breath cycles. This connects the crown and the base of the body.

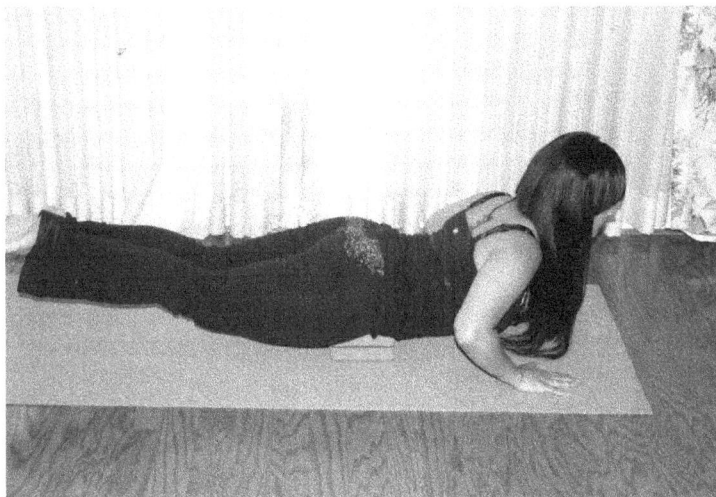

This position works on the ovaries and uterus. It encourages proper blood flow in the pelvis. To get there, place a yoga block at the base of your lower abdomen, lay on it and suspend your body with your arms. Lift your legs so your body weight is on the block and your forearms. While here, take a few deep breaths and ease out of the position. (Do not engage this position while menstruating)

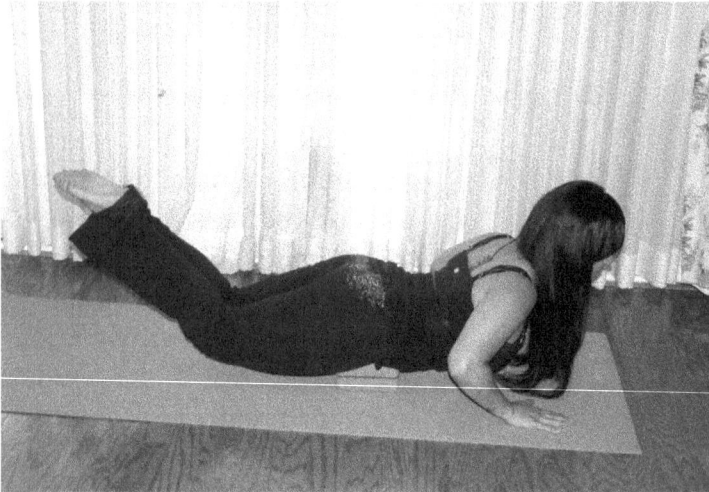

To increase the activation of this area, you may lift your legs up to a 45^0 angle.

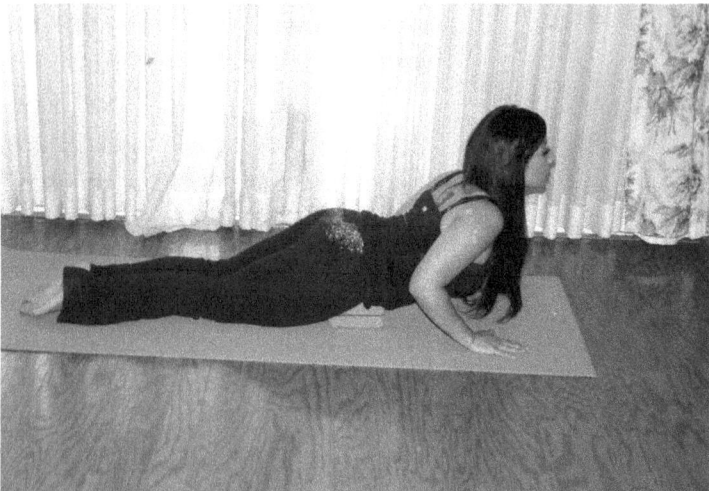

Return to the original position, drop your legs to the floor, take in a deep breath and lift your chest and head. Look ahead of you and rest your palms flat on the mat. Continue to breathe in deeply and exhale through the nostrils.

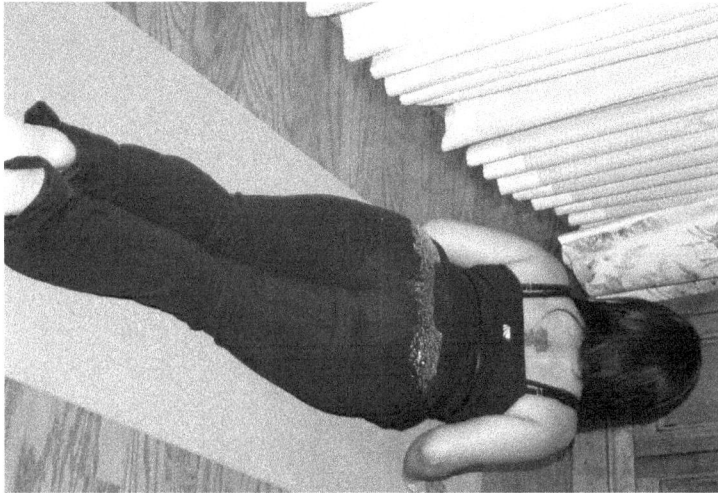

Long view of the above position.

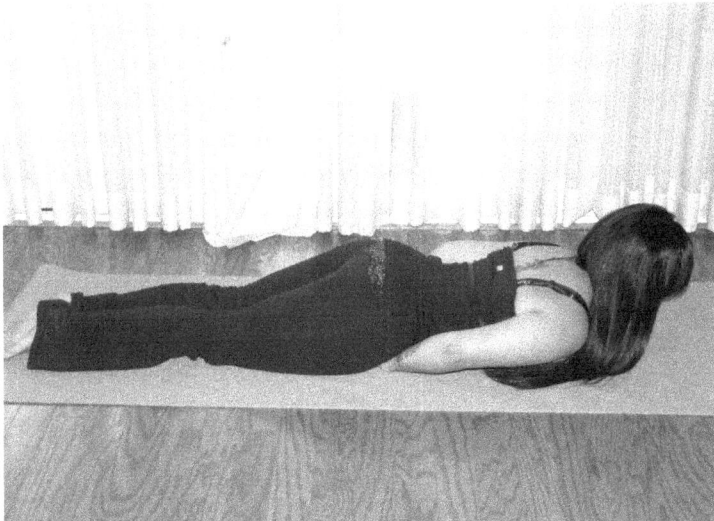

If you do not have a yoga block, or you do not like the feeling of a yoga block against your pelvis, ball up your hands in a fist and place the fists in the grooves of your left and right pelvic joints. Breathe in deeply and exhale fully. Remain in this position for at least 60 breath cycles.

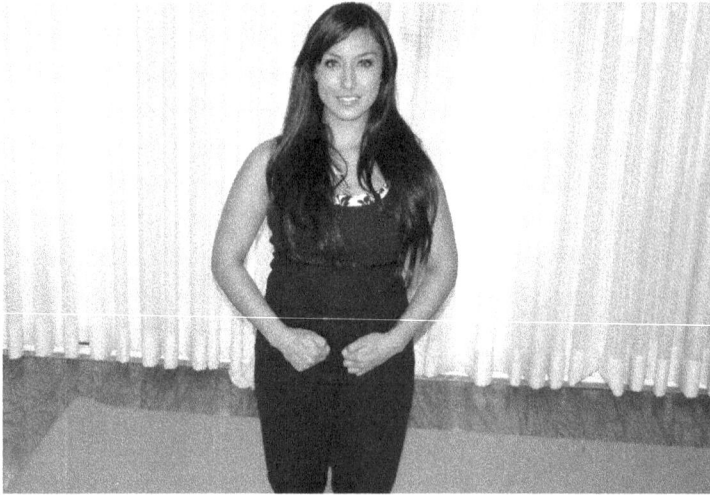

Frontal view of the previous position so you can see where the fists need to be placed.

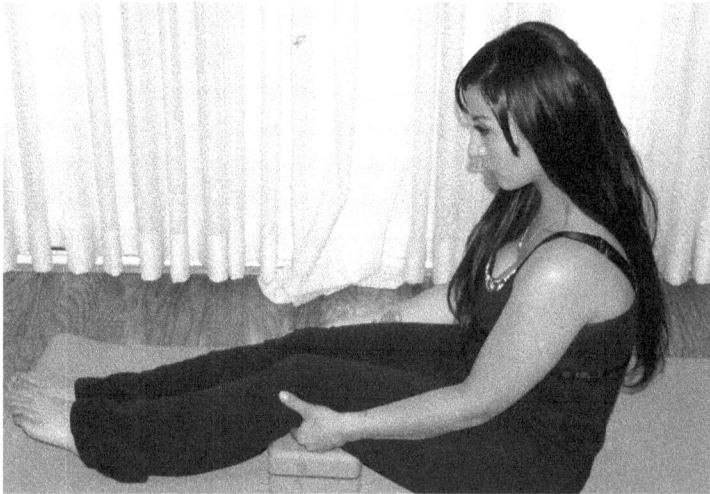

Cup your fingers and place the two middle fingers in the groove of your knee joints. Gently press on this area as you count to 60, release and relax. You may repeat this point pressure for up to 5 times. This point stimulates the lower back and assists in circulation.

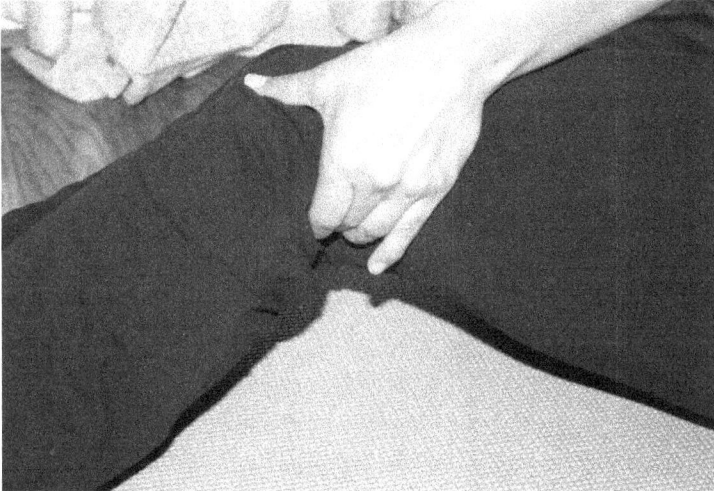

Close up view to show the point being stimulated.

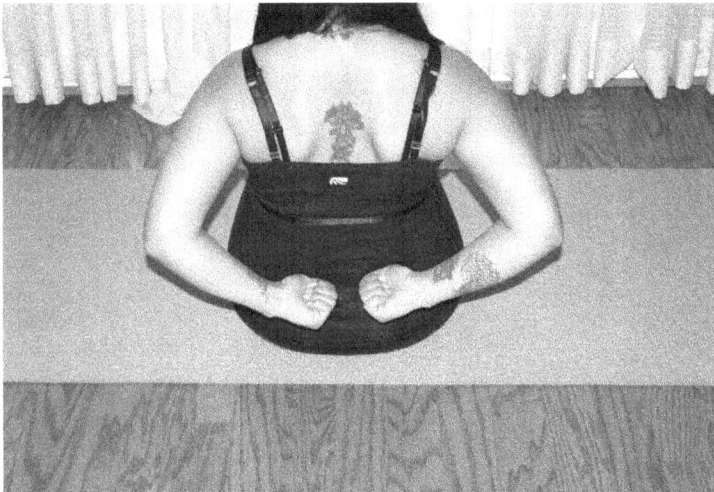

This area of the back has many beneficial points for women's health. You can stimulate some of these points by placing your fists as shown, right on the dimples in the lower back and gently push in. Beneficial for sciatica, low back pain due to PMS or sacral pain. It is also a good relief point after sitting for a long time.

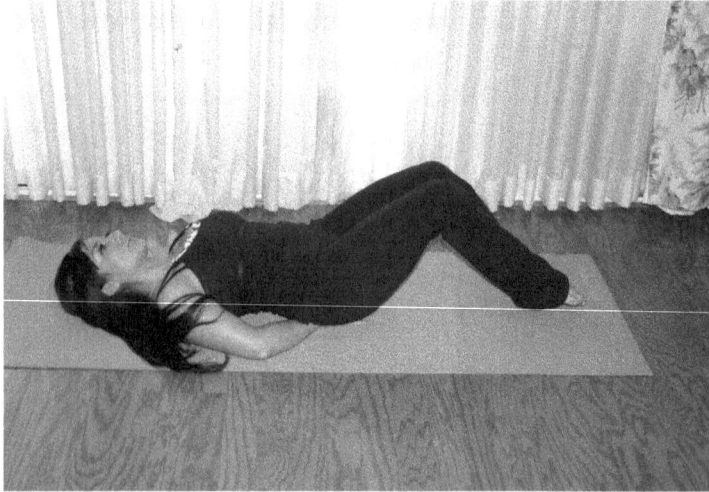

Lay down and gently lift one hip up to place your palm face down on the mat; repeat on the other hip. Adjust your palms so they are cushioning the sides of your tail bone and your bottom is sitting on the back of your palms. Begin to take deep breaths in, hold and release. Repeat for 10 full breath cycles. You are stimulating various sacral points at the same time with this exercise.

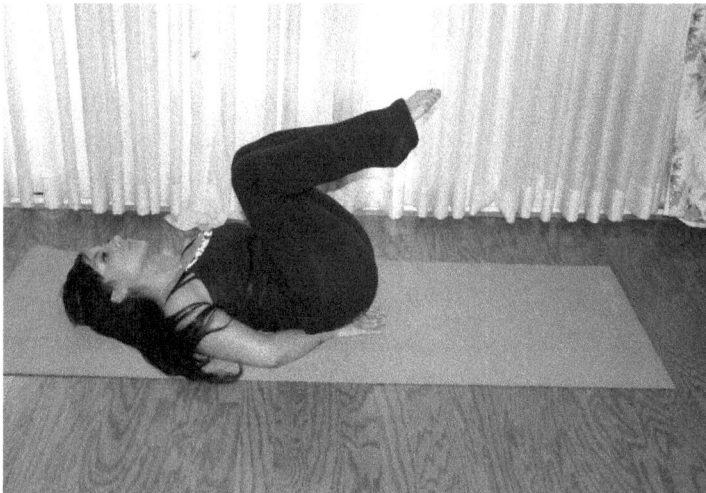

To increase the stimulation at the sacral points, gently lift your legs and take 5 full breath cycles and relax.

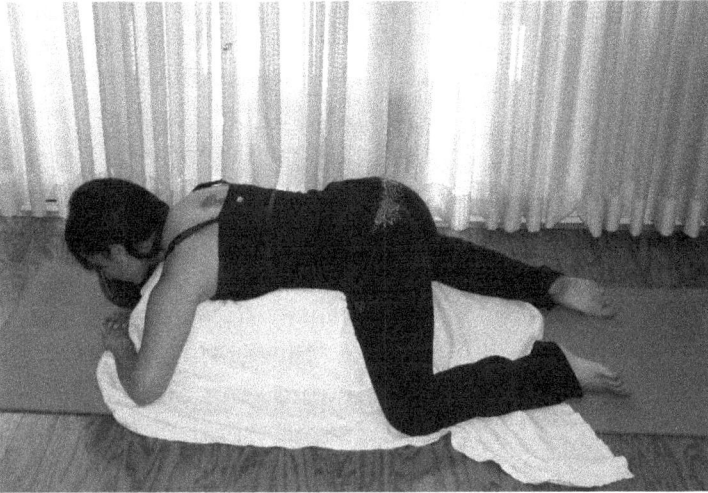

Time to relax a little. To settle into this position, gather a few blankets or pillows and stack them, cover with a sheet as shown. Lay across the stacked blankets and cradle them as shown. Ensure your pelvis is resting at the edge of the stacked blankets or pillows. I like blankets because they provide firm, yet gentle pressure. Relax and breathe in deeply. Stay in this position for 10 – 15 minutes to stimulate circulation, relieve menstrual cramps or abdominal discomfort. This position also helps uro-reproductive problems.

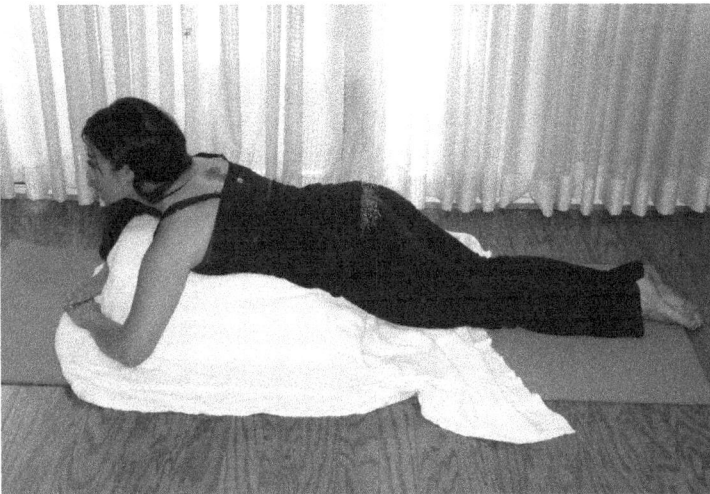

In this position, we are stimulating the same pressure points while encouraging lower back relief. This is excellent if there is low back pressure or sciatic pain accompanying PMS. Straighten your legs and lift your head just above the shoulder. Do not strain neck as you lift. Count to 10, stop to rest and repeat 2 more times.

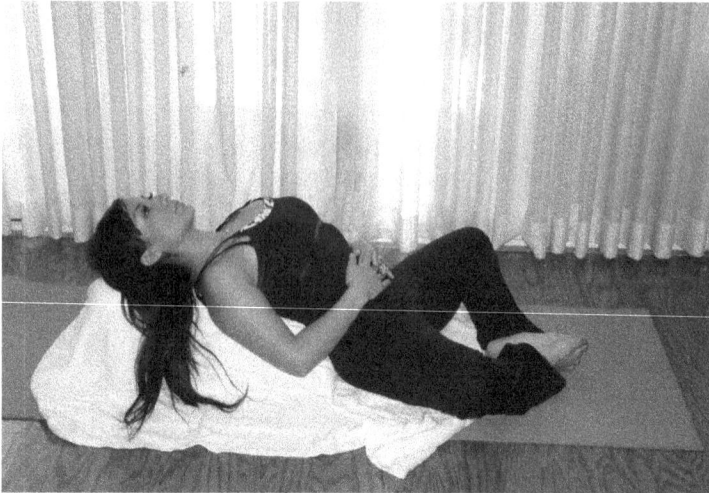

Turn over and sit at the edge of the stacked blankets. Use your hand to support your body as you gently lay back on the blankets. Bring your legs up and together as shown, interlock your fingers and place them over your pelvis. Start to breathe in deeply into your abdomen. As you inhale, send your breath to your pelvis and visualize the breath cleaning out your pelvis and filling it with life. Remain here for 10 – 15 minutes. You may close or open your eyes. I have had clients who chose to pray while in this position, you can do the same if desired. This position helps to open us up to higher spiritual consciousness, stimulate our desire for healthy living, and sustainment of life. This is part of my daily routine and I like to use the time to pray and receive inspiration and deepen my connection with the Divine.

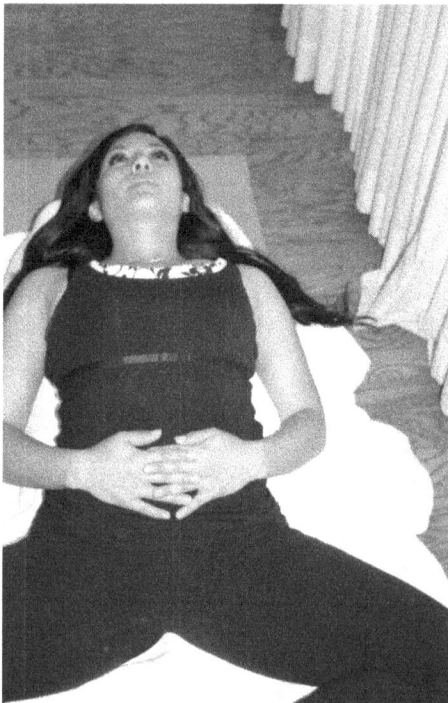

Long view to show placement of hands.

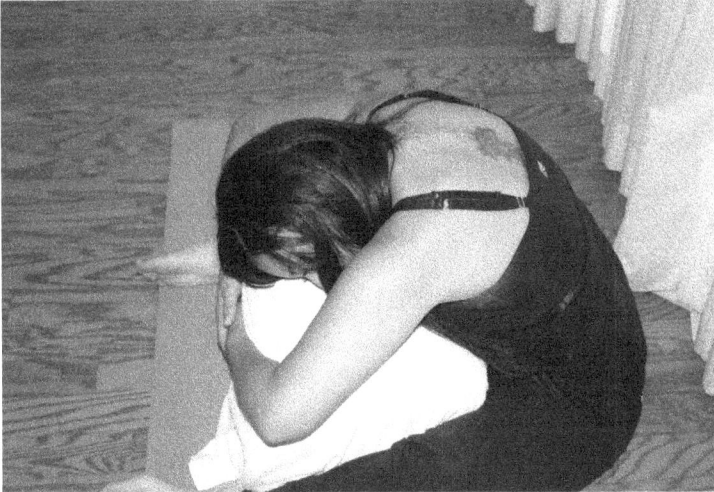

Come to a sitting position, straddle the stacked blankets and rest your head as shown. This position is beneficial for lower abdominal pain or discomfort due to PMS. I call this "the cradle" and I have, on occasion, dozed off in this position.

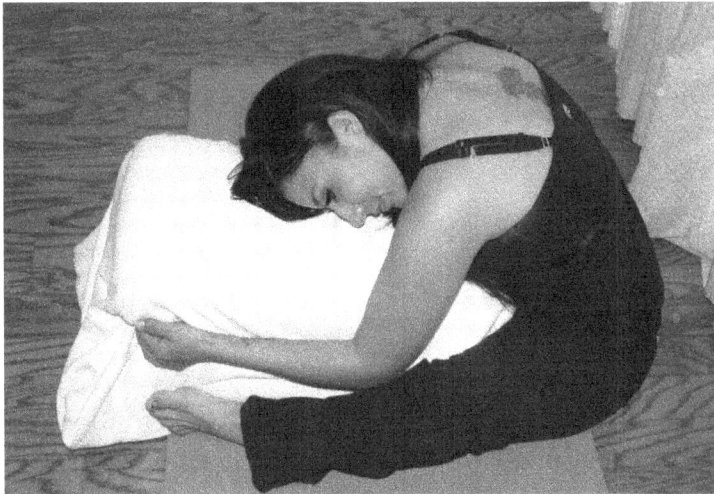

This is the same position with the stacked blankets positioned lengthwise for easy straddling. This is advantageous for those with decreased flexibility in the pelvic joints.

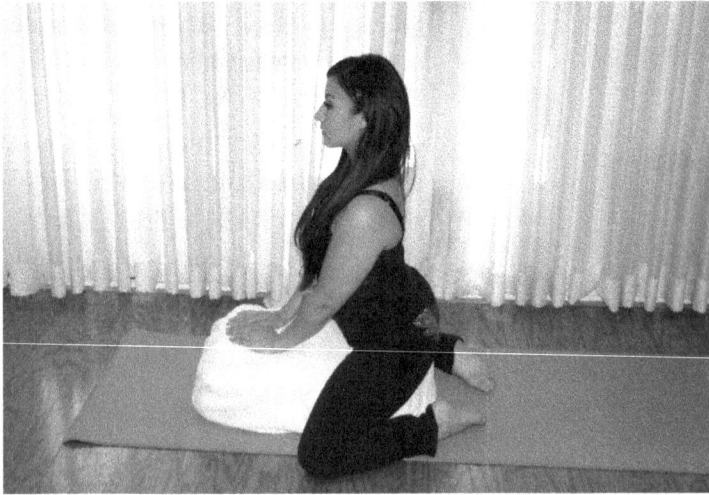

Sit at the edge of the stacked blankets as shown, straighten your spine and bring your palms together before you as shown. Your pelvis should be fully cushioned on the stacked blankets and your abdomen lifted to support the spine. This position encourages proper blood flow to the pelvis and is very beneficial for lower back pain and pelvic joint tightness. Do not force this position.

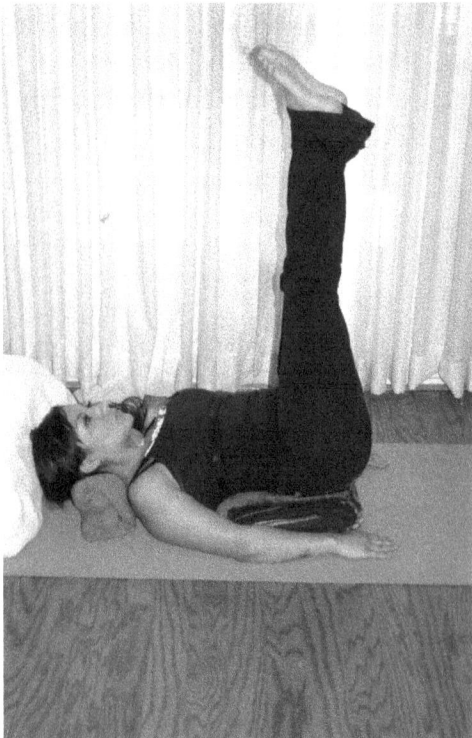

You will need two blankets and a neck pillow or rolled towel for neck support for this position. Stack the two blankets and lay on them as shown. Support your neck with the rolled towel or neck pillow. Gently lift your legs and straighten them as shown. Rest your arms on the mat, palms facing down. Take deep breaths in and slowly count to 15. Fold your legs and plant your feet on the mat, take a deep breath in, relax and straighten your legs to fully come out of the position.

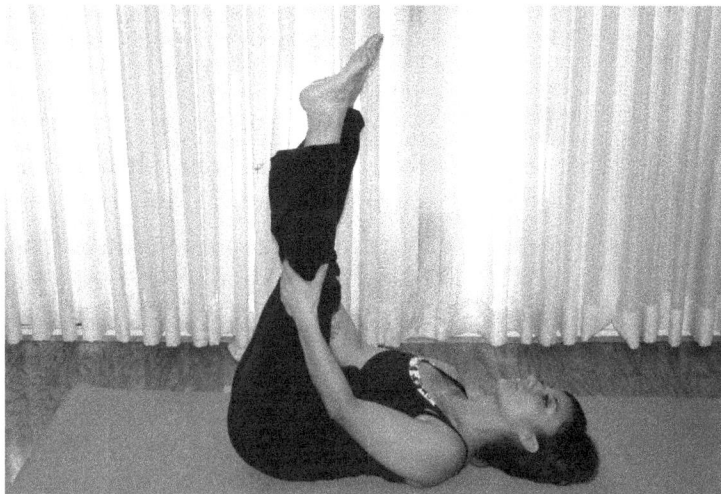

Sit up and remove the stacked blankets and neck support. Lay back down and one after the other, pick up your legs and straighten. Use your arms to support your legs at the knee. Adjust your finger placement to ensure the two middle fingers are touching the knee flex (the point at which your knee folds). Take deep breaths and stay in this position for 60 seconds. This position helps stretch the spine and provide better support for your core.

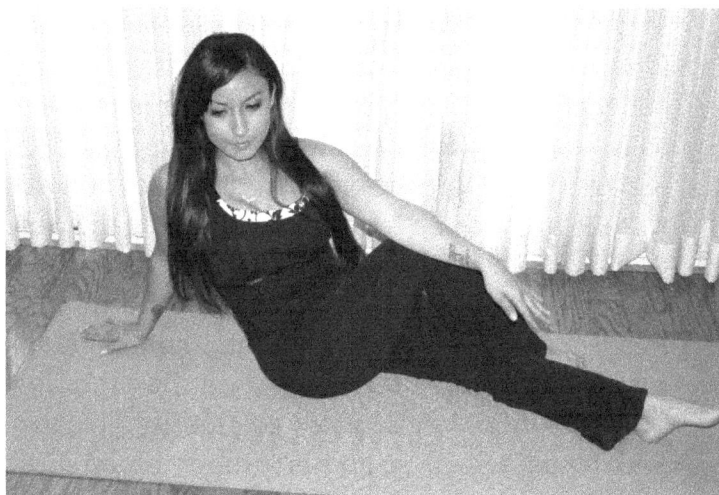

Come to sitting position. Straighten your legs, cross one leg over the other knee as shown. Bring the opposite arm over the bent knee while supporting yur and gently turn your upper body in toward the knee for a gentle stretch. Release and repeat on the other side. This position stimulates the ascending and descending colon and the pelvic region.

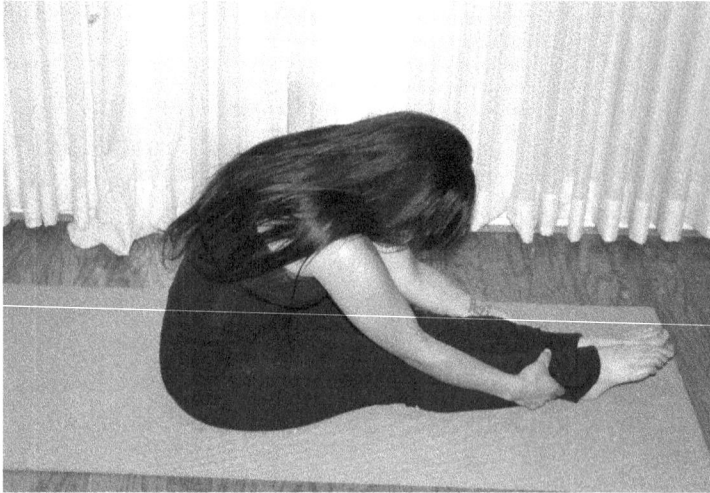

Straighten your legs, start to fold forward as shown and support your upper body with your arms at your ankles (may be exactly at ankles if you can stretch that far or just above the ankle or at the calves if you cannot stretch that far. This position stimulates points at the outer pelvic region and the ovaries (if you have had an oophorectomy, don't worry, do it anyway, you will still benefit)

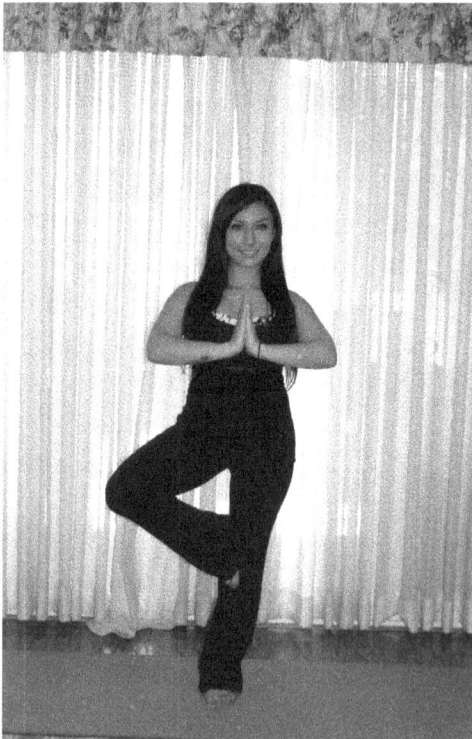

Stand up and plant your feet firmly on the mat. One by one, splay your toes to ensure each toe connects to the mat. Bring your palms together as if you want to pray, slowly pick up your left leg and place it against the right ankle (you can raise it higher to the knee or tucked against the thigh if you can reach that high without wobbling). Take full breath cycles for a minute. Release and plant the left leg into the mat. Relax for a few seconds, then repeat on the other leg. This position helps with grounding, balance and focus which supports proper blood flow and clarity.

Emotional Release Script

(It is better to record this script ahead in your voice and play it to relaxing music. Support yourself with pillows and blankets under your knees to help your back. Turn off all distractions and maintain silence except for the music and your voice aiding you in the session).

Gently allow your eyes to close
Take a deep breath
Relax as you breathe out
Focus on your breathing for a while
Notice how the air is warmer as you breathe out

Start to imagine clouds on a lovely sunny day
See the clouds as you did when you were a child; beautiful, joyous, free, relaxing and enjoyable
Imagine all the beautiful things in the sky
Imagine how it feels to be relaxed because the sky is beautiful
Appreciate how it feels to be relaxed
Appreciate how peaceful it feels

Imagine you are looking at perfect white clouds in the bright blue sky
Start to see the clouds come down and get closer to you
Imagine a fluffy cloud floating down and surrounding you as you relax
The cloud is gently massaging your whole body with soothing healing energy
Your body is starting to loosen and relax
You are feeling safe and secure
The cloud is helping to remove any tension in your body
All areas of tension in your body are being soothed
And you are getting limp and relaxed

Your mind is feeling calm and relaxed and still
Your mind is feeling soothed as the clouds pushes out any negative emotion out of your mind
You are feeling mentally and physically relaxed
You are feeling calm and in control
You are feeling so calm

Continue to feel more relaxed and calm as you breathe in deeply and exhale slowly
You are now beginning to feel peacefulness come over your entire body with each breath you take
As you continue to move deeper into a deep peaceful state
Your subconscious mind begins to review many things that are important to you

It is beginning to look like you are in a library
Your subconscious is a library full of books
These books are about you

Get closer and see all the topics, rows after rows of books about you
From the time your soul began to exist, you have been accumulating knowledge and experiences about you.
Look around in your library and see all your experiences
Good and bad, pleasant and unpleasant, they are here
Move closer to your books
On the right aisle, the books are positive; these are all the beautiful things in your life
On the left aisle, the books hold all the feelings, thoughts, experiences that has caused you negative emotions
Begin to look at the titles; fear, anger, pain, hurt, sorrow, guilt, negativity, nay sayers,
Call each one out by its name
Walk to your anger book, pull it off the shelf and open it
Begin to tear up the pages into tiny pieces and release all your anger
Let it go
As you release anger, see it float away and picked up by a large garbage bin
Tear up your entire anger book and throw it away
Return to your aisle and pick up your fear book
Begin to tear up the pages and release all your fear
Fear of becoming, fear of doing, fear of achieving, fear of the unknown, release them all and dump them in the garbage bin
Next pick up your pain book
This book holds all your pain, all the pain you have ever felt
Begin to tear up each page of this book and release them
Throw the torn pages in the garbage bin
Let your pain go
Release all of the emotions that has caused you pain from this book
Next return to the shelf and pick up your book that contains all the hurt you have ever experienced
Open the book and start to rip out the pages
Tear them up and toss the torn pieces in the garbage
See all your hurt leaving and going into the garbage
Release them and feel freedom from hurting

When you are finished releasing all the things that have hurt you
Return to your shelf and pick up sorrow
Open the book and start to tear up the pages
These pages hold all the sorrow you have experienced in your life
Don't linger or bother to analyze them, simply start to release each sorrowful situation as you tear up the pages of this book
Eliminate sorrow from your life
Release them and throw them into the garbage
On the shelf, you find your book that is holding all the guilt you have experienced
All the instances that have caused you to feel guilty are in this book
Pick it up and open the cover
Start to rip out the pages one by one and tear them into tiny pieces
Tear up all your guilt and throw them in the garbage
Release yourself from all guilt and let them go
Experience freedom from guilt and throw all the pages of guilt away
Go back to your left aisle
You see some other books still on the shelf
One is titled negativity
Pick it up and open it
Rip out the pages of negativity and shred them between your hands
Tear them up, tear up all the negativity you have ever experienced and stored in this book
Release yourself from negativity
Experience freedom and liberation
As you tear up the pages, know that you are free of negativity
Do not bind yourself to this feeling any longer
Let it all go and feel freedom from negativity awash you
Return to the shelf and pick up the book about Nay Sayers
This book holds all the things that you have recorded as impossible
Things you or someone has said you cannot do
Open this book and start to rip out the pages
Tear them up and throw them away
Throw away all your nay sayings and the memories they hold
Remove them from your subconscious and toss them in the garbage
As you throw them away, know that you are free of nay sayings
It does not affect you anymore
You are not a victim of any of these emotions
You are free

Go back to the shelf and find any other negative books it holds
You know them, pick them up and toss them in the garbage
Release your subconscious of these negativities
Toss all the books until there are none left on this aisle

When you finish, push the large garbage bin of all your negativity to the door,
Open the door and toss the garbage in the incinerator
Burn them all and erase them completely
You are no longer beholden to these emotions
You are free

Now look to the right aisle
There are books there with titles of success, positivity
Pick up success and open it
Read the lines congratulating you on every successful thing in your life
See the new sentences of congratulations forming because you have just uncluttered
your subconscious of negative emotions
Feel the exhilarating warmth of success enveloping you
Take some time to read some of the successful events in your life
It could be childhood achievements from school or projects you have accomplished,
Celebrate your successes
Now look up and notice the cloud above you
Take deep breaths in as you watch the cloud

Imagine with each exhale, you are pushing the cloud farther and farther away
The cloud is taking away all your tension and any remnants of negative emotion
And they are moving farther and farther away from you
With each exhalation, you are feeling calmer and deeply relaxed
The cloud is disappearing and you are feeling completely relaxed
You are relaxing mentally and physically

Now imagine your body feeling lighter and lighter
So light you are almost floating
Floating away to a completely safe and relaxing place
Imagine you are slowly starting to float upwards
As you float to the ceiling
Look and observe the difference in your surroundings
Notice the objects in the room

Look at yourself seating peacefully

Start floating out of the ceiling
Out through the roof
Knowing that you are safe as you are floating
Knowing that you are in control
Look around at the streets, the building as you are floating
Float a little higher to a height that is comfortable for you
Look at the area
Notice any familiar places
Any unusual landmarks
Do you see anything that you remember?

Keep floating and float to anywhere you like
It may be anywhere you like
Any where that brings you peace, calmness, serenity
Float to it and enjoy experiencing this peace, this calmness, this serenity
Enjoy drifting around and basking in this peace
Bask in the calmness
Bask in the serenity

Continue to breathe deeply as you are feeling more relaxed, even calmer, more at peace
Welcome any thoughts of bliss and serenity
And let these thoughts bring your warmth and happiness
Look around and see peace, calm, serenity, rest, relaxation, happiness, bliss
They are waiting for you with arms outstretched
Move towards peace and let it wrap its arms around you
Let is surround you and welcome it into your mind and your body
Spend some time soaking up peace as it willingly pours itself into you
Feel it filling you from your toes, to your ankles,
Feel it move upwards to your knees, up to your thighs
Feel peace in your groin, feel it in your abdominal cavity
Feel peace moving upwards to your chest
Feel peace moving up your spine one vertebrae to another
As peace is moving up, feel it filling your lungs and deepening each breath you take
Feel peace in your heart as it hugs your heart completely so that your heartbeats are gentle, normal, and serene

Feel peace moving through your throat, to your mouth, your nose, your eyes
Feel peace hug your ears and move into your brain
Feel peace gently making a nice beautiful home in your brain
As it smiles and whispers that it will always be with you
Thank peace for coming into your life and welcome it whole heartedly into your life

Look around in your peaceful place
You see that peace has brought calm, serenity, rest, relaxation, happiness and bliss with it
Smile and rejoice as you welcome calm, serenity, rest, relaxation, happiness and bliss into your life
Be assured that they travel with peace to help you every time
See them as they beam love and light to you
See the beacon wrap itself around you from your head to your toes
You are completely covered in love and light
You are surrounded by peace, calm, serenity, rest, relaxation, happiness and bliss
You are filled with joy and contentment
You are beaming and radiant
You are calm
You are happy
You are serene
You are relaxed
You are blissful
You are restful
You are peace
You are love
You are light
You are blessed

Meditation Script

First, please note that meditation is not a worship or a prayer; it is a state of awareness. You are paying particular attention to something and observing the experience, when you meditate. The word "meditation" is derived from two Latin words: meditari (to think, to dwell upon, to exercise the mind) and mederi (to heal). Meditation is also a process of freeing yourself from other distractions of the mind and concentrating on that singular activity such as observing your breath or listening to the birds sing. The technique you will learn here is for a beginner and you can do it for as little as 5 minutes a day to get started. So now that you have some clarity about meditation, let's get started.

First, ensure you will not be disturbed by any distractions such as phones, radios, children, husbands, work, etc.

Next, settle into a comfortable position. I encourage you to use pillows, blankets or blocks for additional comfort and support so you are not straining or tensing.

You can light a candle and play some soothing music. Nature sounds are very effective for many people and are great in assisting our minds to settle down and sink into a meditative state.

Once you are comfortable, pick something you like and use it as your focal point. It could be a flower (some of my clients actually use their favorite flowering plants as a focal point), a lit candle (the flame of the candle is the focal point), a photo of your favorite spiritual being, a favorite word, or affirmation.

Begin to breathe in deeply and exhale fully as you start to concentrate on your focal point.

You may notice your thoughts wandering while you are trying to concentrate, don't focus on them or try to control your thoughts. Simply allow them to flow in and out while you maintain focus on your focal point. You are an observer, observe your thoughts with detachment, and do not process them.

Keep your focus on the point and continue to breathe.

After a few minutes, shift your focus to your breathing and observe your inhalation and exhalation.

Gently come out of this state and remain sitting for a while. Whenever you are ready, conclude by brushing your hands over your eyes and down your face and bring your palms together before your heart center.

Resources

For more health and wellness information, products and services, visit,
www.drabiola.com
Herbs: www.mountainroseherbs.com
　　　www.banyanbotanicals.com
Supplements: www.supplementdirect.com
Environmental Working Group: www.ewg.org
Organic Consumers Association: www.oca.org

Bibliography

Balch, P. A. (2000). *Prescription for nutritional healing.* (3rd ed.). NY: Avery.

Barnard, N. D. (2001). Turn off the fat genes: The revolutionary guide to losing weight. NY: Three Rivers Press.

Best, G. F. (2000). *Secrets of healing with nutrition and herbs: Research-based recommendations for health.* San Antonio, TX: Self Published.

Carlson, N. R. (2004). *Physiology of behavior* (8th ed.). Boston: Allyn and Bacon.

Fishbein, M., & Fishbein, J. (Eds.). (1978). *Fishbein's illustrated medical and health encyclopedia.* NY: Stuttman Company Inc.

Gerras, C., Hanna, J. E., Feltman, J., Bingham, J, Golant, J., & Moyer, A. (Eds.) (1976). *The encyclopedia of common diseases.* NY: Rodale Press.

Ghizzani, A., Razzi, S., Fava, A., Sartini, A., Picussi, K., & Petraglia, F. (2003). Management of sexual dysfunctions in women. *Journal of Endocrinological Investigation.* 26(3 Suppl), 137-8.

Hawkes, S., Morison, L., Foster, S., Gausia, K., Chakraborty, J., Peeling, R.W., & Mabey, D. (1999). Reproductive-tract infections in women in low-income, low-prevalence situations: assessment of syndromic management in Matlab, Bangladesh. *The Lancet.* 354 (9192), 1776-1781.

Human Anatomy Online. (2010). *The female reproductive system.* Retrieved from http://www.innerbody.com/image/repfov.html

Jensen, B. (1993). *Foods that heal: A guide to understanding and using the healing powers of natural foods.* NY: Avery.

Jensen, B. (2000). *Dr. Jensen's guide to body chemistry and nutrition.* Lincolnwood, IL: Keats Publishing.

Jensen, B. (2000). *Dr. Jensen's nutrition handbook: A daily regimen for healthy living.* Lincolnwood, IL: Keats Publishing.

Kalat, J. W. (2004). *Biological psychology* (8th ed.). Belmont, CA: Wadsworth/Thomson Learning.

Komaki , K., Ohno, Y., & Aoki, N. (2005). Gonadal hormones and gonadal function in type 2 diabetes model OLETF (Otsuka Long Evans Tokushima Fatty) rats. *Endocrine Journal.* 52(3), 345-51.

Lee, J. R., Hanley, J., & Hopkins, V. (1999). *What your doctor may not tell you about premenopause: Balance your hormones and your life from thirty to fifty.* NY: Time Warner Books.

Lee, J. R., Zava, D., & Hopkins, V. (2002). *What your doctor may not tell you about breast cancer: How hormone balance can help save your life.* NY: Time Warner Books.

Martire, M., Pistritto, G., & Preziosi, P. (1989). Different regulation of serotonin receptors following adrenal hormone imbalance in the rat hippocampus and hypothalamus. *Journal of Neural Transmission,* 78(2), 109-20.

McDougall, J. A. (1990). The McDougall Program: 12 days to dynamic health. NY: Penguin Books.

Nagaoka, T., Onodera, H., Matsushima, Y., Todate, A., Shibutani, M., Ogasawara, H. & Maekawa, A. (1990). Spontaneous uterine adenocarcinomas in aged rats and their relation to endocrine imbalance. *Journal of Cancer Research and Clinical Oncology,* 116.

National Institute of Health. (n. d.) *Endocrine System (Hormones).* Retrieved August 17, 2010 from http://health.nih.gov/search.asp/7

Nilsson, R. (2000). Endocrine modulators in the food chain and environment. *Toxicologic Pathology*, 28(3), 420-31.

Parch, L. (2006). The nine best herbs for women. *Natural Health*, 36(8), 74-79.

Physicians Committee for Responsible Medicine. (2002). *Healthy eating for life for women.* NY: John Wiley & Sons, Inc.

Pinel, J. P. K. (2003). *Biopsychology.* (5th ed.). Boston: Allyn and Bacon.

Rustia, M. (1979). Role of hormone imbalance in transplacental carcinogenesis induced in Syrian golden hamsters by sex hormones. *National Cancer Institute Monograph*, 51, 77-87.

Sarrel, P.M. (1990). Ovarian hormones and the circulation. *Maturitas*, 12(3), 287-98.

Savitz, D. A., Whelan, E. A., & Kleckner, R. C. (1989). Self-Reported Exposure to Pesticides and Radiation Related to Pregnancy Outcome: Results from National Natality and Fetal Mortality Surveys. *Public Health Reports*, 104, 473-477

Siddiqi, M. A., Laessig, R. H., & Reed, K. D. (2003). Polybrominated diphenyl ethers (PBDEs): new pollutants-old diseases. *Clinical medicine and research.* 1(4), 281-90.

Starr, C. & Taggart, R. (1995). *Biology: The unity and diversity of life.* (7th ed.). Belmont, CA: Wadsworth/Thomson Learning.

Steiner, M., & Pearlstein, T. (2000). Premenstrual dysphoria and the serotonin system: pathophysiology and treatment. *The Journal of Clinical Psychiatry*. 61(12 Suppl), 17-21.

Steiner, M., & Born, L. (2000). Advances in the diagnosis and treatment of premenstrual dysphoria. *Adis* 13(4), 287-304.

Vanderhaeghe, L. R. (2004). *An A-Z woman's guide to vibrant health: Prevent and treat the top 25 female health conditions*. Hillsburgh, ON: Health Venture Publications.

Walraven, G., Scherf, C., West, B., Ekpo, G., Paine, K., Coleman, R., Bailey, R., & Morison, L. (2001). The burden of reproductive-organ disease in rural women in The Gambia, West Africa. *The Lancet*, 357 (9263), 1161-1167.

Warshowsky, A. & Oumano, E. (2002). *Healing Fibroids: A doctor's guide to a natural cure*. NY: Fireside.

www.ingramcontent.com/pod-product-compliance
Lightning Source LLC
Chambersburg PA
CBHW081157270326

41930CB00014B/3189